DIALYSIS

NURSING CARE

THE COMPLETE GUIDE

ALEXANDRE CAREWELL

Table of Contents

« Nephrology is not just about understanding the kidneys, but about capture the very essence of life filtered drop by drop. »

INTRODUCTION

My career as a dialysis nurse

More than two decades ago, when I was finishing my nursing studies, I could never have imagined the extent to which the speciality of dialysis would transform my professional and personal life. It's a story of passion, dedication, challenge and constant learning. This is my journey through the fascinating world of dialysis.

• My beginnings in the world of health
It all started in a general hospital where I was assigned to different wards in my first year of practice. There I met patients with all sorts of illnesses, from newborn babies to the elderly. However, one ward in particular caught my attention: the nephrology ward. I was struck by the resilience of renal failure patients and the complexity of the care needed to support them. I realised that each dialysis session was not just a medical procedure, but a delicate dance between technology, nursing expertise and the well-being of the patient.

• Diving into dialysis
My interest in nephrology led me to seek specialist training in dialysis. I joined a renowned centre, where I was trained by some of the best professionals in the field. Every day was a mixture of technical challenges, rapid clinical decisions and profound human interaction. I learned to understand the dialysis machines, but more than that, I learned to understand the patients who depended on them.

• Challenges and rewards

Dialysis, although vital, is not without complications. I have witnessed difficult times, when patients have suffered complications or become discouraged by the constant routine of sessions. But with these challenges have come priceless moments of triumph. Seeing a patient recover after a crisis, helping a family understand the dialysis process, or simply sharing a smile with a patient during a difficult session has made the journey rewarding.

• Continuous learning

The field of nephrology is constantly evolving. New techniques and technologies emerge regularly, requiring nurses to keep up to date and adapt their skills. Over the years, I've attended many conferences, taken part in training courses and even contributed to research to continue to improve patient care.

• Reflections

Today, looking back, I'm filled with gratitude for the experiences I've had and the lives I've been able to touch. Dialysis is more than a medical procedure; it's a chance to give life back, session after session. For anyone thinking of entering this field, know that it is a demanding but deeply rewarding journey.

This journey as a dialysis nurse has shaped not only my career, but also my outlook on life. Every patient, every challenge and every success has reminded me of the inestimable value of health, determination and, above all, human empathy.

Why dialysis is essential

Dialysis, a word that many people associate with medical complexity, lies at the crossroads of cutting-edge technology and human compassion. But why is it so crucial? To answer this question, we first need to understand the fundamental nature of the kidneys and their vital role in the human body.

1. THE KIDNEYS: OUR NATURAL PURIFIERS
The kidneys are two bean-shaped organs located on either side of the spine, just below the rib cage. Their main role is to filter the blood to eliminate waste and excess fluid, transforming this waste into urine. In other words, they act as our body's natural purifiers, ensuring that harmful substances are eliminated effectively.

2. RENAL FAILURE: WHEN PURIFIERS BREAK DOWN
Sometimes the kidneys do not work properly or stop working altogether. This can be due to a variety of reasons, ranging from genetic diseases to acquired conditions such as hypertension or diabetes. When the kidneys lose their ability to filter blood effectively, waste products accumulate in the body, leading to a series of dangerous symptoms such as fatigue, loss of appetite, nausea and swollen extremities.

3. DIALYSIS: A LIFE-SAVING REMEDY
This is where dialysis comes in. It acts like an artificial kidney, taking over when the natural kidneys can no longer do their job. Dialysis allows the blood to be filtered outside the body, eliminating waste and excess fluid, then returned to the patient purified.

4. A LIFELINE FOR MANY PATIENTS
Without dialysis, patients with end-stage renal disease would see toxins accumulate in their bodies, which could

quickly become fatal. For many, dialysis is literally a lifeline, allowing for increased quality of life and life expectancy despite severely compromised kidney function.

5. BEYOND FILTRATION: ELECTROLYTE AND HORMONE BALANCE

The kidneys are not only responsible for filtration. They also play a key role in the balance of electrolytes in the body and the production of certain essential hormones. Dialysis also helps to regulate this balance, ensuring that levels of substances such as potassium and sodium remain within healthy limits.

Dialysis is much more than just a medical procedure. It is a bridge to life for those whose kidneys are not functioning properly. It represents the fusion of science and medicine, offering a chance of survival and improved quality of life to thousands of people every day. For carers, patients and their families, understanding the vital importance of dialysis is the first step to successfully navigating the journey of kidney failure.

Who is this book for?

When I set out to write this guide to dialysis, my ambition was not simply to provide a technical overview. On the contrary, I wanted to provide a comprehensive, accessible and practical resource capable of meeting the varied needs of a wide range of readers. So, who exactly is this book for?

1. FUTURE HEALTHCARE PROFESSIONALS
- **Nursing students:** This book is an ideal introduction for those who are just starting out on their nursing course and want to familiarise themselves with the speciality of dialysis.

- **Entry-level nurses :** For those who have just joined a dialysis department or are considering doing so, this guide provides a comprehensive and in-depth overview of the procedures, techniques and best practices of the profession.
- **Other healthcare professionals:** Doctors, technicians and other medical professionals who work with dialysis teams will also benefit from this book to better understand the process and improve interdisciplinary patient management.

2. PATIENTS AND THEIR FAMILIES
- **Dialysis patients:** Although this book is technical, some chapters may help patients to understand the dialysis process, the issues involved and the importance of treatment compliance.
- **Families and loved ones:** Understanding what their loved ones are going through can be both reassuring and enlightening. This book provides valuable information to help families support and accompany their loved ones through their dialysis journey.

3. EDUCATORS AND TRAINERS
Teachers, trainers and other health educators will find this book an excellent teaching aid. It can be used as a reference manual, to supplement a curriculum or as part of ongoing training.

4. FOR THOSE WHO ARE CURIOUS AND PASSIONATE ABOUT MEDICINE
For those who have always been fascinated by the medical world and wish to deepen their knowledge of a specific subject, this book offers a detailed and accessible overview of dialysis, its importance and how it works.
Conclusion
My dearest wish is that this book will become an invaluable resource for everyone who reads it. May it be a beacon of

light for professionals navigating the sometimes tumultuous waters of dialysis, a source of comfort for patients and their families, and a well of knowledge for everyone else.

Chapter 1:
UNDERSTANDING DIALYSIS

What is dialysis?

• History and development of dialysis

Dialysis may seem like a modern invention, but its roots run deep in the history of medicine. The evolution of this technology and the theories surrounding it is a fascinating testament to human ingenuity, innovation and the eternal imperative to save lives. Here is an overview of the history and development of dialysis.

1. THE BEGINNINGS: THE PRINCIPLES OF DIFFUSION AND OSMOSIS

- **The concept of dialysis:** The term "dialysis" comes from the Greek "dia", meaning "through", and "lysis", meaning "dissolution" or "separation". It describes the process of separating solutes through a semi-permeable membrane.
- **Early discoveries:** Thomas Graham, a 19th century Scottish chemist, is often called the "father of dialysis". In 1861, he discovered the principle of diffusing solutes through a membrane, which he called "dialysis".

2. THE FIRST ATTEMPTS

- **First machines:** In the 1910s, the first dialysis machines were designed, but they were rudimentary and ineffective in treating kidney failure.
- **Innovation during the war: It** was during the Second World War, faced with large numbers of wounded suffering from acute renal failure, that the first functional dialysis machines were developed, notably

by Dr Willem Kolff, considered to be the "father of modern dialysis".

3. THE MODERN DIALYSIS REVOLUTION

- **Kolff rotary dialyser:** In 1943, Willem Kolff developed the first rotary dialyser using cellophane tubes. This was a turning point, leading to the first successful cure of a patient in 1945.
- **Peritoneal dialysis:** In the 1950s and 1960s, doctors began experimenting with peritoneal dialysis, in which the patient's peritoneum serves as the dialysis membrane.
- **Technological advances:** The 1970s and 1980s saw huge advances in dialysis technology, with the introduction of machines that were safer, more efficient and more comfortable for patients.

4. DIALYSIS TODAY

- **Home haemodialysis:** Technological advances have made it possible for many patients to receive haemodialysis at home, increasing their comfort and independence.
- **Biocompatibility and biomimetics:** Current research is focusing on developing more biocompatible membranes to reduce adverse reactions and improve dialysis efficiency.
- **Research into artificial kidneys:** The quest for a portable or implantable artificial kidney is one of the Holy Grails of nephrology research.

From the simple observation of natural phenomena to today's cutting-edge medical technology, the history of dialysis is a testament to human determination to overcome challenges and improve quality of life. Every innovation, every discovery has been guided by a profound desire to help those suffering from kidney failure, making dialysis a true celebration of science and humanity.

• The different forms of dialysis

Although often perceived as a uniform procedure, dialysis actually comes in several forms, each adapted to specific needs and offering its own advantages and disadvantages. These forms have evolved over the years, responding to both technological advances and the clinical requirements of patients. Let's explore the main forms of dialysis.

1. HAEMODIALYSIS (HD)

This is the most widespread form of dialysis and the one most familiar to the general public.

- **Principle:** The patient's blood is pumped out of the body, filtered through a dialyser (or artificial kidney) to remove waste and excess fluid, then returned to the body.
- **Advantages:** Effective, controlled in a hospital environment, allows close monitoring of the patient.
- **Disadvantages:** Generally requires long sessions several times a week, can be restrictive for the patient, risk of infection at the vascular access site.

2. HOME HAEMODIALYSIS (HDD)

A variation on traditional haemodialysis that allows patients to undergo dialysis at home.

- **Principle:** Similar to standard haemodialysis, but carried out at home using specially adapted equipment.
- **Benefits:** Greater flexibility, more frequent but shorter dialysis periods, improved quality of life.
- **Disadvantages:** Requires extensive training, the creation of an appropriate home environment, and the responsibility of the patient or a carer to administer the treatment.

3. PERITONEAL DIALYSIS (PD)

- **Principle:** The peritoneum, a natural membrane in the abdomen, is used as a filter. A dialysis solution is introduced into the abdominal cavity and, after a certain amount of time, is drained off, taking with it waste products and excess fluid.

- **Advantages:** Can be performed at home, greater freedom for the patient, no need for heavy machinery, longer preservation of residual renal function.
- **Disadvantages:** Risk of peritoneal infection, requires several fluid exchanges a day or a machine for automated peritoneal dialysis at night.

4. HEPATIC DIALYSIS

Less common and used mainly for acute liver failure.

- **Principle:** Similar to haemodialysis, but designed to eliminate toxic substances that accumulate as a result of liver failure.
- **Benefits:** Potentially lifesaving for patients waiting for a liver transplant or recovering from severe hepatitis.
- **Disadvantages:** Less common, requires specialist equipment.

The choice between these different forms of dialysis will depend on many factors, including the patient's general state of health, lifestyle, personal preferences and geographical location. It is vital that patients and healthcare professionals work closely together to identify the most appropriate and effective method for each individual.

• Dialysis as a renal replacement

The kidneys play a vital role in maintaining the body's homeostatic balance, filtering waste products and excess fluid and excreting them in the form of urine. When the kidneys can no longer perform this vital function, dialysis becomes an essential alternative. Let's take a look at dialysis as a kidney replacement.

1. MAIN FUNCTIONS OF THE KIDNEYS

- **Filtration and elimination:** The kidneys filter around 120 to 150 litres of blood each day to produce around 1 to 2 litres of urine, eliminating waste and excess substances.
- **Fluid balance:** They regulate the volume and concentration of different body fluids.
- **Electrolyte regulation:** The kidneys maintain the balance of electrolytes such as sodium, potassium and calcium.
- **Hormone production:** They produce hormones that influence other bodily functions, such as the production of red blood cells (erythropoietin) and the regulation of blood pressure (renin).

2. THE NEED FOR A RENAL SUBSTITUTE

- **Acute renal failure (ARF):** A sudden deterioration in renal function, often reversible with appropriate management.
- **Chronic renal failure (CRF):** A progressive and often irreversible deterioration in kidney function, requiring long-term management.

3. HOW DIALYSIS IS USED AS A KIDNEY SUBSTITUTE

- **Elimination of waste:** Like a natural kidney, dialysis eliminates waste and excess substances from the blood.
- **Balancing electrolytes:** Dialysis helps regulate levels such as potassium, sodium and bicarbonate, to maintain a stable electrolyte balance.
- **Elimination of excess fluid:** By removing excess fluid, dialysis helps prevent oedema, hypertension and other complications associated with fluid overload.
- **Helps regulate blood pressure:** By maintaining an appropriate volume and fluid balance.

4. LIMITATIONS OF DIALYSIS AS A RENAL REPLACEMENT

- **Not an exact copy:** Although dialysis imitates many kidney functions, it cannot completely replace a natural, functioning kidney.
- **Lack of hormone production:** Dialysis machines cannot produce hormones in the same way as natural kidneys.
- **Frequency and duration:** Dialysis sessions are generally required several times a week and may last several hours, unlike natural kidneys, which work continuously.

Although dialysis is essential for many people suffering from kidney failure, it never completely replaces the function of a healthy kidney. It acts as a bridge, prolonging life and improving quality of life, while waiting for a possible kidney transplant or recovery of kidney function. Understanding the capabilities and limitations of dialysis enables patients to be better managed and care to be tailored to individual needs.

Why do some patients need dialysis?

• Acute renal failure

Acute renal failure, also known as acute kidney injury, is a condition in which the kidneys suddenly stop working properly, failing to filter waste products from the blood. This condition can progress in a matter of hours or days and can be potentially fatal if not treated promptly. Let's take a closer look at this condition.

1. CAUSES OF ARI

ARI can be caused by a multitude of factors, generally classified into three main categories:

- **Pre-renal:** Problems affecting blood flow to the kidneys.
    - Dehydration
    - Shock (hypovolaemic, cardiogenic)
    - Medications that affect renal blood supply, such as NSAIDs
    - Cardiac disorders
- **Renal (or intrinsic):** Problems directly related to the kidneys.
    - Glomerulonephritis
    - Nephrotoxic drugs (such as certain antibiotics)
    - Autoimmune diseases
    - Kidney infections
    - Renal vascular diseases
- **Post-renal:** Obstructions affecting the evacuation of urine.
    - Kidney stones
    - Prostate hypertrophy
    - Tumours
    - Urinary tract obstructions

2. SYMPTOMS OF ARI

Symptoms may vary depending on the severity of the condition and the underlying cause:
- Reduced urine production
- Water retention, causing swelling of the legs, ankles or feet
- Shortness of breath
- Fatigue
- Confusion
- Nausea
- Irregular heartbeat

3. DIAGNOSIS

The diagnosis is generally based on :
- Patient's medical history and symptoms
- Blood tests to measure creatinine and urea

- Urine analysis
- Ultrasound or other imaging tests

4. TREATMENT
Treatment depends on the cause of the ARF:
- **Treatment of the underlying cause:** For example, stopping a nephrotoxic drug or treating an infection.
- **Management of symptoms and complications:** This may include medication to balance electrolyte levels, diuretics to increase urine production or other treatments to manage specific symptoms.
- **Dialysis:** In serious cases where the kidneys do not recover their function quickly, temporary dialysis may be necessary to replace the filtration function of the kidneys.

5. PREVENTION
Although not all causes of ARI can be prevented, certain preventive measures can reduce the risk:
- Adequate hydration, particularly during intense physical activity or in hot weather.
- Cautious use of medicines, particularly those that may affect renal function.
- Regular health checks for people at risk.

Acute renal failure is a medical emergency requiring rapid intervention. With early diagnosis and appropriate management, kidney function can often be restored. The key is rapid recognition of symptoms and immediate medical intervention.

• Chronic renal failure
Chronic kidney disease (CKD) is a progressive and usually irreversible loss of kidney function. It occurs when the kidneys are damaged and can no longer filter blood as effectively as before. Let's take a closer look at this disease.

1. CAUSES OF CKD

A number of conditions can lead to CKD, including :

- **Diabetes:** This is the most common cause of CKD. Excess sugar in the blood can damage the nephrons, the filtration units of the kidneys.
- **Hypertension:** Uncontrolled high blood pressure can cause damage to the blood vessels in the kidneys.
- **Glomerulonephritis:** Inflammation of the glomeruli, which are the small filtration units in the kidneys.
- **Hereditary diseases:** such as polycystic kidney disease.
- **Urinary obstructions:** such as kidney stones or prostatic hypertrophy.
- Autoimmune diseases: such as lupus.

2. SYMPTOMS OF CKD

Symptoms are often subtle and can develop slowly over several years. They include:

- Fatigue and weakness
- Shortness of breath
- Swelling of the ankles, feet and hands
- Persistent itching sensation
- Frequent urination, especially at night
- Hypertension
- Loss of appetite
- Sleep disorders
- Nausea or vomiting
- Concentration problems

3. DIAGNOSIS

Diagnosis is based on :

- **Blood tests:** Measurement of creatinine and urea levels.
- **Urinalysis:** Evaluation of proteins and other abnormalities.
- **Medical imaging:** ultrasound, MRI or CT scan to visualise the kidneys.

- **Kidney biopsy:** A small sample of kidney tissue is taken to be examined under the microscope.

4. TREATMENT
Although CKD often cannot be reversed, it is possible to manage the condition and slow its progression:
- **Controlling the underlying causes: For example,** managing diabetes or hypertension.
- **Medication:** To treat symptoms and complications, such as diuretics, antihypertensives or drugs to regulate electrolyte levels.
- **Dietary changes:** Limiting protein, salt and other minerals can help reduce the workload on the kidneys.
- **Dialysis:** When the kidneys can no longer function properly, dialysis may be necessary to replace their filtration function.
- **Kidney transplantation:** This is an option for certain patients, where a healthy kidney from a donor replaces a diseased kidney.

5. PREVENTION
Prevention is based on managing the underlying conditions and maintaining a healthy lifestyle:
- Regular monitoring of blood pressure and blood sugar levels.
- Maintain a healthy weight.
- Adopt a balanced diet.
- Limit alcohol consumption and avoid smoking.
- Avoid non-essential nephrotoxic drugs.

Chronic kidney disease is a serious medical condition with potentially serious health implications. With early detection, appropriate management and lifestyle changes, it is possible to slow its progression and effectively manage symptoms. Awareness of CKD is crucial to ensure early management and improved quality of life for patients.

• Other indications for dialysis

Although chronic and acute renal failure are the main reasons why dialysis is commonly used, there are other medical conditions and situations that may require dialysis. Here is an overview of other indications for dialysis:

1. INTOXICATION AND OVERDOSE

- **Medication:** Certain drugs, such as barbiturates, lithium and aspirin, can cause dialysis if taken in overdose.
- **Toxins: In** the case of intoxication by certain substances, dialysis can help remove the toxin from the system, as with ethylene glycol (antifreeze) or methanol.

2. ELECTROLYTE IMBALANCE

- **Severe hyperkalaemia:** A high concentration of potassium in the blood can be fatal, affecting heart function. Dialysis can be used to rapidly eliminate excess potassium.
- **Severe imbalances in other electrolytes:** Such as very high levels of calcium or phosphate.

3. SEVERE METABOLIC ACIDOSIS

When the body produces an excess of acids or cannot eliminate them properly, this can lead to acidosis. In some cases, the kidney cannot restore the acid-base balance, necessitating dialysis.

4. WATER OVERLOAD

In some patients, particularly those with heart failure, the body's ability to eliminate excess fluid may be compromised, leading to fluid overload. If diuretics are not effective, dialysis may be necessary to eliminate this excess fluid.

5. MYELOMA SYNDROMES

In some cases of multiple myeloma, large quantities of light proteins (light chains) are produced, which can damage the kidneys. Dialysis can help remove these proteins from the blood.

6. AUTOIMMUNE DISEASES

In conditions such as systemic lupus erythematosus, where there is an abnormal production of antibodies that can damage the kidneys, dialysis may be necessary, especially during a severe flare-up of the disease.

7. OTHER SYSTEMIC DISEASES

Certain diseases, such as scleroderma or vasculitis, can have an impact on kidney function. In advanced cases or in the presence of complications, dialysis may be a treatment option.

Although kidney failure remains the most common indication for dialysis, it is also used as a vital treatment in a number of other medical situations. Understanding these indications enables healthcare professionals to act quickly when a patient could benefit from a dialysis procedure. Dialysis's ability to rapidly filter blood of various substances makes it essential in a wide range of clinical settings.

Chapter 2:
THE DIALYSIS ENVIRONMENT

Organisation of the dialysis department

Running a dialysis department requires meticulous organisation to ensure patient safety, provide quality care, optimise resources and guarantee the well-being of professionals. Here's how a dialysis department is generally organised:

1. SERVICE STRUCTURE
- **Dialysis rooms:** These areas are equipped with chairs or beds for patients, as well as dialysis machines, monitoring equipment and other essential equipment.
- **Reception area:** to register patients on arrival, manage their appointments and direct them to the dialysis room.
- **Preparation areas:** These areas are dedicated to the preparation of dialysis solutions and the necessary equipment.

2. DEPARTMENT STAFF
- **Specialist dialysis nurses:** They play a central role in the running of sessions, monitoring patients, preparing machines and managing any complications.
- **Nephrologists:** Kidney specialists who supervise treatment, adjust dialysis parameters and treat medical complications.
- **Dialysis technicians:** They prepare and maintain the machines, make sure the equipment is working properly and sometimes help out during sessions.

- **Social assistants:** They provide support for non-medical aspects, such as counselling, referral to resources or management of social and financial problems.
- **Dieticians:** They advise patients on appropriate diets for dialysis and help them to manage dietary restrictions.
- **Administrative staff:** They manage administrative aspects such as booking appointments, billing and coordination with other medical services.

3. PROTOCOLS AND PROCEDURES

- **Admission procedures:** Initial patient assessment, creation of medical records, planning of dialysis schedule.
- **Safety protocols:** These define measures to prevent infection, manage medical waste, guarantee sterilisation of equipment and ensure the safety of patients and staff.
- **Ongoing training:** Regular programmes for staff to keep them up to date with the latest techniques, research and safety standards in dialysis.

4. INTERDISCIPLINARY COLLABORATION

- **Regular meetings:** These meetings between nephrologists, nurses, technicians, dieticians and social workers allow patients' cases to be examined, challenges to be discussed and care to be coordinated.
- **Liaison with other services:** collaboration with radiology services for arteriovenous fistulas, with surgery for kidney transplants or with psychology for emotional support.

5. **CONTINUOUS IMPROVEMENT**
- **Patient feedback:** Surveys or interviews to understand patient experience and suggest improvements.
- **Internal audit:** Regular review of processes, patient outcomes and standards of care to identify areas for improvement.

Organising a dialysis service is a complex task requiring close coordination between many professionals and constant attention to the safety and quality of care. A well-managed service not only improves patient outcomes but also contributes to their general well-being and that of the professionals who care for them.

Equipment required for a dialysis session

• Dialysis machines
The dialysis machine is at the heart of dialysis treatment. Its design and function are essential for purifying the blood of patients suffering from kidney failure. This section explores the structure, operation and maintenance of these machines.

1. MACHINE STRUCTURE AND COMPONENTS
- **Monitor:** Displays dialysis parameters such as blood flow, elapsed time, dialysis solution volume and other essential information.
- **Blood pump:** Regulates the circulation of the patient's blood through the dialyser.
- **Dialyzer:** Also known as an "artificial kidney", this is where the exchange between the patient's blood and the dialysis solution takes place.

- **Dialysis solution pumps:** Control the flow of dialysis solution through the dialyser.
- **Heating system:** heats the dialysis solution to an appropriate temperature before it reaches the dialyser.
- **Alarm system:** Warns of anomalies or malfunctions.

2. HOW IT WORKS
- **Preparing the machine:** Before each session, the machine is prepared, making sure that all the components are working properly and that the necessary solutions are ready.
- **Blood circulation:** Blood is drawn from the patient, usually through a vascular access such as a fistula, and then pumped through the dialyser.
- **Purification:** In the dialyser, the blood is separated from the dialysis solution by a semi-permeable membrane. Waste products and excess fluid are transferred from the bloodstream to the dialysis solution, which is then drained off.
- **Blood return:** After passing through the dialyser, the purified blood is returned to the patient.

3. CARE AND MAINTENANCE
- **Daily cleaning:** After each session, the machine is cleaned to prevent infection and ensure optimum performance.
- **Disinfection:** The machines are regularly disinfected to eliminate any microbial contamination.
- **Regular maintenance:** Components such as pumps and alarm systems are checked and serviced regularly to ensure they are working properly.
- **Replacing parts: Over** time, some parts may wear out and need to be replaced to ensure safe and effective treatment.

4. INNOVATIONS AND TECHNOLOGICAL ADVANCES

- **Portable machines:** New compact machines allow patients to receive dialysis at home or on the move.
- **Customisation:** Technological advances mean that dialysis parameters can be further personalised for each patient.
- **Integration technologies:** Modern machines can often be integrated with other hospital systems, allowing remote monitoring and management.

Dialysis machines are complex and vital devices that require constant attention and meticulous maintenance. Understanding their structure and operation is essential for any professional working in a dialysis department. As technology advances, these machines continue to evolve, offering improved care to patients suffering from kidney failure.

• Supplies and consumables

In the dialysis setting, it is crucial to have the right supplies and consumables to ensure safe and effective patient care. These items are generally single-use to prevent infection and ensure sterility. Here is an overview of the supplies and consumables commonly used in a dialysis department:

1. VASCULAR ACCESS

- **Catheters:** Used for temporary or permanent access, they are inserted into large blood vessels.
- **Needles:** Specially designed for arteriovenous fistulas and grafts.
- **Bandages and dressings:** To cover and protect the access site after dialysis.

2. DIALYZER AND CIRCUITS

- **Disposable dialysis machines:** Also known as "artificial kidneys", these contain a semi-permeable membrane to filter the blood.

- **Tubing:** Tubing that connects the patient to the dialysis machine.
- **Rinsing solutions:** To prepare and test the circuit before dialysis.

3. DIALYSIS SOLUTIONS
- **Bags of concentrated solution:** are mixed with purified water to create the dialysis solution.
- **Bicarbonate acid:** Often used to adjust the pH of the dialysis solution.

4. MEDICINES AND ANTICOAGULANTS
- **Heparin:** Prevents blood clotting during dialysis.
- **Medication to treat complications:** Such as antihypertensive drugs, calcium solutions or anti-nausea drugs.

5. CLEANING AND DISINFECTION SUPPLIES
- **Disinfectant solutions:** For cleaning machines and surfaces.
- **Sterile wipes:** For cleaning access sites or areas of the skin.

6. TEST SUPPLIES
- **Test strips:** For checking water quality and solution concentration.
- **Blood sampling kits:** For monitoring electrolyte levels, kidney function and other important parameters.

7. MISCELLANEOUS ITEMS
- **Disposable gloves:** For protection and infection prevention.
- **Medical waste bags:** For safe disposal of used consumables.

- **Syringes and needles:** For administering medicines or taking samples.

8. PERSONAL PROTECTIVE EQUIPMENT (PPE)
- **Gowns:** Protect staff from accidental contact with blood or solutions.
- **Masks and goggles:** Protect against splashes.
- **Caps and overshoes:** To maintain a sterile environment.

Dialysis supplies and consumables play an essential role in ensuring that treatment is not only effective but also safe for patients and healthcare staff. The management of these consumables requires rigorous organisation, appropriate storage and ongoing training for staff to ensure their correct and effective use.

Health and safety standards

Hygiene and safety are of paramount importance in a dialysis department. Dialysis patients are often immunocompromised and at increased risk of infection. In addition, the dialysis process involves direct exposure to blood, increasing the risk of disease transmission. Here is an overview of the essential health and safety standards in the context of dialysis:

1. HAND HYGIENE
- **Regular hand washing:** Before and after each patient, before and after wearing gloves, and after any contact with body fluids.
- **Use of alcohol-based disinfectants:** In addition to washing hands with soap and water.

2. PERSONAL PROTECTIVE EQUIPMENT (PPE)

- **Gloves:** Change between patients and after any contact with blood or other body fluids.
- **Gowns, masks, goggles:** To be worn during procedures where there is a risk of splashing.
- **Handling and disposal:** Properly remove and dispose of PPE to avoid cross-contamination.

3. DISINFECTION AND STERILISATION

- **Surfaces:** Regularly clean and disinfect surfaces, especially those in direct contact with the patient or equipment.
- **Dialysis machines:** Follow the manufacturer's specific instructions for cleaning and disinfection.
- **Reusable instruments:** Sterilise according to medical standards after each use.

4. WASTE MANAGEMENT

- **Specific containers:** Use containers specifically designed for biomedical waste.
- **Safe disposal: Ensure** that waste is collected and disposed of in accordance with regulatory standards.

5. PATIENT SAFETY

- **Education:** Patients must be informed about the risks, benefits and procedure of dialysis.
- **Monitoring:** Constant monitoring of patients during dialysis to detect any problems at an early stage.

6. STAFF SAFETY

- **Training:** Staff must be regularly trained in health and safety best practice.
- **Vaccinations:** Ensure that all staff are up to date with the necessary vaccinations, in particular hepatitis B.

7. INFECTION PREVENTION

- **Water control:** The water used for dialysis must be regularly tested and treated to eliminate contaminants.
- **Preventing infections linked to vascular access:** Use aseptic techniques for the insertion and maintenance of catheters, fistulas and grafts.8. Emergencies
- **Emergency equipment:** Have emergency equipment available, such as a defibrillator, emergency kit and oxygen.
- **Emergency protocols:** Staff must be trained to react quickly to emergencies such as falls, allergic reactions or cardiovascular complications.

Hygiene and safety standards in dialysis are essential to protect both patients and staff. They require constant vigilance, regular training and updating in line with new research and recommendations. By complying with these standards, dialysis services can offer high-quality care while minimising the risks for everyone.

Chapter 3:
THE ROLE OF THE DIALYSIS NURSE

Preparing the patient

• Clinical evaluation

Clinical assessment is a fundamental part of the management of dialysis patients. It is used to determine the patient's general state of health, the effectiveness of dialysis and the possible presence of complications or new pathologies. Here is a detailed guide to the clinical assessment of a dialysis patient:

1. QUESTIONING
- **General symptoms:** Fatigue, weight loss, fever, nausea, vomiting or any other unusual symptoms.
- **Specific symptoms:** Cramps, itching, shortness of breath, oedema, hypertension or hypotension, pain at the vascular access site.
- **Medication:** All current medications, recent changes, drug allergies and side effects.
- **Medical history:** Previous illnesses, surgeries, hospitalisations and other medical treatments.

2. PHYSICAL EXAMINATION
- **Vitality:** Measurement of blood pressure, heart rate, respiratory rate and temperature.
- **Vascular access site:** Check for redness, swelling, heat or pain. Listen for blood flow sounds (thrill) to confirm proper function.
- **Cardiovascular examination:** Listen to heart sounds, check for oedema in the legs, assess peripheral circulation.

- **Lung examination:** Listen to the lungs for wheezing, rales or other abnormal sounds.
- **Abdominal examination:** Palpate to detect any mass, pain or distension.

3. LABORATORY ASSESSMENTS
- **Blood tests:** Measure levels of urea, creatinine, electrolytes, bicarbonate, haemoglobin and other important indicators to assess renal function and the effectiveness of dialysis.
- **Urine tests:** to check for the presence of protein, blood or other abnormalities.
- **Other specific tests:** For example, parathyroid hormone levels for patients with secondary hyperparathyroidism.

4. QUALITY OF LIFE ASSESSMENTS
- **Emotional and mental states:** Depression, anxiety or other psychological problems common in dialysis patients.
- **Activity level and functional capacity:** Assess the patient's ability to carry out daily activities.

5. NUTRITIONAL ASSESSMENT
- **Weight:** Monitor weight fluctuations to assess fluid balance.
- **Dietary intake:** Examine the diet to ensure that it is suited to the kidney condition.

6. PERIODIC ASSESSMENTS
- **Regular reassessment:** Patients should be assessed regularly to monitor their progress and adjust treatment if necessary.
- **Consultations with other specialists:** as required, for example, a cardiologist, endocrinologist or psychologist.

Clinical assessment is an ongoing process that requires attention to detail, active listening and close collaboration with the patient. It enables problems to be detected early, treatment to be adjusted and comprehensive care to be provided, optimising outcomes for dialysis patients.

• Psychological preparation

Dialysis is a major transition for most patients. Beyond the physical implications, dialysis can have a profound emotional and psychological impact. Psychological preparation is therefore essential to help patients manage this new phase in their lives.

1. RECOGNISING THE EMOTIONAL IMPACT

- **Lifestyle changes:** Include changes to daily routine and commitment to treatment.
- **Fears and anxieties:** Acknowledge concerns about the procedure, the future and changes in health.
- **Feelings of loss:** Identify feelings of loss of normal kidney function and independence.

2. EMOTIONAL SUPPORT

- **Support groups:** Direct patients to support groups where they can share their experiences and learn from others.
- **Individual therapy:** For those who need it, therapy can help deal with feelings of depression, anxiety or bereavement.
- **Family and friends:** Encourage patients to talk about their feelings and concerns with those close to them.

3. EDUCATION AND INFORMATION

- **Dialysis process:** Explaining in detail what to expect during dialysis can help reduce anxiety.
- **Symptom management:** Information on how to manage common side effects, such as fatigue, cramps or low blood pressure.

- **Patient rights:** Reassuring patients of their rights, including the right to participate in decision-making about their treatment.

4. STRESS MANAGEMENT TECHNIQUES
- **Relaxation:** teaching patients techniques such as deep breathing, meditation and guided visualisation.
- **Physical activity:** Encourage appropriate physical activity to reduce stress and improve mood.
- **Hobbies and recreational activities:** Motivating patients to pursue or find new hobbies to distract and relax.

5. PREPARING FOR ROUTINE CHANGES
- **Planning:** Helping patients to plan their timetable to fit in dialysis sessions.
- **Adapting to the workplace:** Discuss possible arrangements with your employer, such as flexible working hours.

6. ENCOURAGING AUTONOMY
- **Training for self-dialysis:** Some patients may choose home self-dialysis options. Training them properly can increase their sense of independence.
- **Active participation:** Encourage patients to ask questions and take an active part in their treatment.

7. CONTINUOUS MONITORING
- **Regular follow-up:** Plan regular consultations with a psychologist or counsellor to monitor the patient's emotional and psychological state.

Psychological preparation is a crucial aspect of managing dialysis patients. Recognising and addressing the emotional and mental challenges associated with dialysis can improve patient quality of life and increase compliance with treatment. A holistic approach that encompasses emotional support, education and stress management is essential to support patients throughout their dialysis journey.

Setting up and dialysis monitoring

• Connecting and disconnecting

One of the most technical stages in the dialysis process is connecting and disconnecting the patient to and from the dialysis machine. This procedure, which requires precision and vigilance, is essential to ensure patient safety. Here is a detailed overview of these steps:

1. PREPARATION
- **Checking equipment:** Make sure all consumables are available: dialysis lines, dialysate solution, anticoagulants, dressings, sterile gloves, etc.
- **Checking the machine: Make** sure that the dialysis machine is clean, in working order and ready for the session.
- **Patient preparation:** Check the vascular access site for signs of infection or complication.

2. CONNECTION
- **Hand washing:** This is a crucial step in avoiding contamination.
- **Preparing the access site:** Clean the vascular access site with a suitable antiseptic and allow to dry.
- **Connection:** Connect the dialysis lines to the machine. Ensure that air is completely removed from the lines to avoid gas embolism.
- **Needle insertion:** If the patient is using a fistula or graft, insert the needles in accordance with the

protocols. If the patient is using a catheter, connect it to the lines.

- **Start dialysis: Once** everything is connected correctly, start the dialysis process by following the prescribed parameters.

3. MONITORING

- **During dialysis:** Monitor the patient continuously for signs of discomfort, hypotension or other complications.
- **Machine monitoring: Make sure** that the machine is operating correctly and that the alarms are activated.

4. DISCONNECT

- **Stopping the machine:** When the session is over, stop the dialysis machine and monitor the patient's vital signs.
- **Removing needles:** Gently remove the needles from the fistula or graft, applying gentle pressure to avoid bleeding.
- **Catheter disconnection:** If a catheter is used, disconnect it from the dialysis lines.
- **Cleaning the site:** Clean the access site again with an antiseptic.
- **Dressing:** Apply a sterile dressing to the access site.

5. AFTER DIALYSIS

- **Post-dialysis monitoring:** Monitor the patient for a period of time to ensure that there are no post-dialysis complications.
- **Advice to the patient:** Tell the patient what to look out for when they get home and when they should come back for the next session.

Connecting and disconnecting the dialysis machine are vital steps that require in-depth training, skill and constant attention. When carried out correctly, these procedures guarantee patient safety and effective treatment.

• Continuous monitoring

Adequate and continuous monitoring is essential during dialysis sessions to ensure patient safety and optimise treatment results. Here is a detailed overview of continuous monitoring during dialysis treatment:

1. MONITOR VITAL SIGNS

- **Heart rate:** Ensure that the heart rate remains within a normal range for the patient. Variations may indicate a complication.
- **Blood pressure:** Abrupt changes in blood pressure may occur during dialysis, particularly due to the rapid removal of fluids.
- **Temperature:** An increase in temperature may indicate an infection.
- **Breathing:** Watch the rate and depth of your breathing. Shallow or rapid breathing may signal a problem.

2. OBSERVATION OF VASCULAR ACCESS

- **Appearance:** Check the access area regularly for signs of infection, redness, swelling or haematoma.
- **Blood flow:** Ensure that blood flow is stable and that there are no signs of obstruction or complications.

3. MONITORING THE DIALYSIS MACHINE

- **Parameters:** Ensure that all parameters (such as dialysate flow rate, temperature, pressure, etc.) are as prescribed for the patient.
- **Alarms:** Make sure all alarms are working properly. In the event of an alarm, quickly identify the cause and take action if necessary.

4. ASSESSMENT OF PATIENT WELL-BEING
- **General symptoms:** Ask patients regularly about their condition, particularly if they experience dizziness, nausea, cramps or any other discomfort.
- **Emotional state:** Make sure the patient is relaxed and reassured. Increased anxiety or emotional distress can have harmful effects.

5. MONITORING WEIGHT AND FLUID BALANCE
- **Weight:** Weigh the patient before and after each session to assess the amount of fluid removed.
- **Urinary volume:** If the patient is still producing urine, measure and document the volume.

6. MONITOR DIALYSATE QUALITY
- **Concentration:** Make sure that the dialysate solution has the correct concentration of electrolytes.
- **Temperature:** Make sure it stays within the prescribed range.

7. ASSESSMENT OF POST-DIALYSIS SYMPTOMS
- **Common symptoms:** After dialysis, some patients may experience fatigue, cramps or headaches. Monitor these symptoms and inform the doctor if necessary.

8. DOCUMENTATION
- **Patient record:** Record all relevant details of the session, including machine settings, vital signs, incidents or complications, and any procedures performed.

Continuous monitoring is a key element in the safety and effectiveness of dialysis treatment. The nurse or technician must be trained to recognise warning signals quickly and intervene appropriately. Careful monitoring not only ensures the patient's physical well-being, but also contributes to their peace of mind during this essential procedure.

Complication management

• Hypotension

Hypotension, or low blood pressure, is one of the most common complications of dialysis, particularly haemodialysis. A thorough understanding of this complication is crucial to its prevention and management.

1. DEFINITION AND DIAGNOSIS
- **What is hypotension?** A decrease in systolic blood pressure below 90 mmHg or a decrease of more than 20 mmHg compared with the patient's initial pressure.
- **Signs and symptoms:** Fatigue, dizziness, nausea, cramps, visual fog, palpitations, chest pain and, in severe cases, loss of consciousness.

2. CAUSES OF HYPOTENSION IN DIALYSIS
- **Rapid withdrawal of fluid:** Withdrawing too much blood volume in a short space of time can reduce blood volume and cause hypotension.
- **Cardiac dysfunction:** Patients with a history of heart problems may have a reduced ability to compensate for rapid changes in volume.
- **Dialysate temperature:** A dialysate that is too hot can cause vasodilation, lowering blood pressure.
- **Antihypertensive medication:** Taking antihypertensive medication before dialysis may increase the risk of hypotension.
- **Meals before dialysis:** Eating just before or during dialysis can direct blood flow to the gastrointestinal tract, reducing blood return to the heart.

3. PREVENTION

- **Adjusting the volume of liquid to be withdrawn:** Accurately estimate the volume of liquid to be withdrawn during each session.
- **Monitoring dialysate temperature:** Keep dialysate at an appropriate temperature to minimise vasodilation.
- **Medication management:** Review and adjust antihypertensive medication before dialysis.
- **Advice on meals:** Advise patients to avoid eating just before or during dialysis.

4. MANAGEMENT OF HYPOTENSION

- **Interrupt fluid removal:** Stop or reduce fluid removal as soon as hypotension is detected.
- **Patient positioning:** Place the patient in the Trendelenburg position (head lower than the feet) to increase venous return.
- **Administration of fluids:** Administer a saline solution to increase blood volume.
- **Continuous monitoring:** Monitor vital signs closely until they stabilise.
- **Assessment of medication:** Reassess the patient's medication, particularly antihypertensive medication, and adjust accordingly.

Hypotension during dialysis is a common but manageable complication. Careful monitoring, prompt intervention and thorough patient education on preventive measures are essential to ensure patient safety and well-being during dialysis sessions.

• Cramps

Muscle cramps are a common complication during haemodialysis. They are often painful and can considerably affect patients' quality of life. Understanding cramps during dialysis and knowing how to prevent and manage them is essential to ensure patient comfort.

1. DEFINITION AND DIAGNOSIS

- **What is a cramp?** An involuntary, sudden and painful contraction of a muscle or group of muscles.
- **Areas affected:** Although any muscle can be affected, cramps during dialysis most commonly affect the leg muscles.

2. CAUSES OF CRAMP IN DIALYSIS

- **Rapid fluid removal**: Rapid fluid removal during haemodialysis can reduce blood volume and electrolyte concentration, causing cramps.
- **Electrolyte imbalance:** Abnormal levels of certain electrolytes, particularly sodium, potassium and calcium, can lead to cramps.
- **Accumulation of toxins:** Dialysis may not eliminate all toxins effectively, which may affect muscle function.

3. PREVENTION

- **Moderate fluid withdrawal:** Make sure you withdraw the prescribed volume of fluid at a moderate rate, avoiding too rapid a withdrawal.
- **Electrolyte monitoring:** Keep an eye on the patient's electrolyte levels and adjust the dialysate if necessary.
- **Taurine supplementation:** Some studies suggest that taurine may help prevent cramps during dialysis, although further research is needed.

4. CRAMP MANAGEMENT

- **Reducing fluid withdrawal:** If the patient begins to cramp, consider reducing the rate of fluid withdrawal.
- **Stretching the affected muscle:** Ask the patient to gently stretch the affected muscle. For example, for a calf cramp, the patient can try stretching their leg and gently pulling their toes towards them.

- **Electrolyte supplements:** If electrolyte imbalance is suspected, consider dialysate adjustment or supplementation.
- **Medication:** In some cases, medicines such as quinine or other antispasmodics may be prescribed, although their use can have side effects.

Cramps during dialysis can be uncomfortable and disruptive for patients. Careful monitoring, prompt intervention and thorough patient education on cramp prevention and management can help improve the dialysis experience and quality of life.

• Other common complications
Although dialysis is a life-saving procedure, it is associated with a series of potential complications. In addition to low blood pressure and cramps, other complications can arise during or after a dialysis session.

1. INFECTION
- **Vascular access:** Access (fistula, graft or catheter) is a potential route for infection.
- **Prevention:** Ensure aseptic technique during connection and disconnection. Monitor access regularly for signs of infection.
- **Management: If there are** signs of infection, treatment may include antibiotics and, in some cases, surgery to remove an infected catheter.

2. ANAEMIA
- **Cause:** Blood loss during sessions and reduced production of erythropoietin by diseased kidneys can lead to anaemia.
- **Prevention:** Minimise blood loss during dialysis and monitor haemoglobin and haematocrit levels regularly.

- **Management:** Administration of erythropoietin and iron supplements if necessary.

3. BONE AND MINERAL PROBLEMS
- **Cause:** Kidney disease can affect the balance of calcium and phosphorus, affecting bones.
- **Prevention:** Controlled diet, phosphorus-binding drugs and dialysate adjustment.
- **Management:** Calcium supplements, active vitamin D and other medicines to regulate bone metabolism.

4. DIALYSIS EXHAUSTION SYNDROME
- **Cause:** Fatigue after dialysis due to rapid changes in body volume and electrolyte balance.
- **Prevention:** Adjusting the rate and amount of fluid withdrawal.
- **Management:** Rest and, in some cases, adjustment of the dialysis schedule.

5. VASCULAR ACCESS MALFUNCTION
- **Cause:** Blockages, stenosis or thrombosis can affect the fistula, graft or catheter.
- **Prevention:** Regular monitoring of access, aseptic techniques and avoidance of compression.
- **Management:** Surgical or radiological interventions to restore circulation.

6. COMPLICATIONS ASSOCIATED WITH THE DIALYSATE
- **Cause:** Electrolyte imbalances, contamination or allergic reactions.
- **Prevention:** Checking the composition of the dialysate and regular maintenance of the dialysis machine.
- **Management:** Adjustment of dialysate and treatment of symptoms.

Knowledge of the potential complications associated with dialysis is essential for their prevention and management. Constant monitoring, open communication with the patient and ongoing education are crucial to ensure patient safety and well-being during and after each dialysis session.

Patient education

Educating patients undergoing dialysis is essential for their autonomy, safety and the success of their treatment. Appropriate information can help patients to better understand their condition, adhere to treatment and play an active role in managing their health.

1. INTRODUCTION TO DIALYSIS
- **What is dialysis?** Explanation of the basic principles.
- **Why is it necessary?** Discussion of kidney function and the reasons for dialysis.
- **Types of dialysis:** Haemodialysis vs. peritoneal dialysis.

2. UNDERSTANDING RENAL FAILURE
- **What do the kidneys do?** The importance of the kidneys in the body.
- Causes of renal failure: Acute vs. chronic.
- **Signs and symptoms:** How to recognise problems.

3. VASCULAR ACCESS
- **Types of access:** Fistula, graft, catheter.
- **Access care:** Hygiene, monitoring and prevention of complications.

4. TYPICAL DIALYSIS SESSION
- **Before the session:** Preparations and expectations.

- **During the session:** Process, monitoring and management of symptoms.
- **After the session:** Recovery, monitoring and home care.

5. DIET AND FLUIDS
- **The importance of diet:** The impact of diet on dialysis and kidney health.
- **Fluid limits:** Importance and management tips.
- **Electrolytes to watch out for:** Potassium, phosphorus, calcium, sodium.

6. MEDICINES
- **Common medications:** Antihypertensives, iron supplements, phosphorus binders.
- **Importance of membership:** Consequences of non-membership.
- **Managing side effects:** How to recognise them and what to do.

7. COMPLICATION MANAGEMENT
- **Recognition:** Signs and symptoms of common complications.
- What should be done in the event of complications? First aid and when to seek help.

8. DAILY LIFE AND EMOTIONAL SUPPORT
- Daily activities: Work, sport, leisure.
- **Emotional support:** Managing stress, depression and anxiety.
- **Available resources:** Support groups, therapies, social services.

9. FUTURE PROSPECTS
- **Kidney transplantation:** What you need to know and how to prepare.

- New technologies and treatments: Keeping abreast of the latest advances.

Patient education is a central pillar in the management of kidney failure and dialysis. By providing patients with the tools and information they need, healthcare professionals can help them lead healthier, more independent and more fulfilling lives.

Chapter 4:
SPECIAL TECHNIQUES

Haemodialysis

• Basic principles

Dialysis is a complex but essential process that partially replaces the function of the kidneys when they can no longer do their job. For a novice patient, or for anyone who wants to understand this procedure, it is crucial to know its basic principles.

1. WHAT IS DIALYSIS?

- **Definition:** Dialysis is a medical procedure that helps remove waste, salt and excess water from the body. It also helps regulate safe levels of certain essential chemicals in the blood, such as potassium, sodium and bicarbonate.
- **Objective: The** main function of dialysis is to maintain the balance of substances in the blood, which the diseased kidneys can no longer do effectively.

2. WHY IS THIS NECESSARY?

- **Role of the kidneys:** The kidneys filter and eliminate waste products from the blood to form urine. They also help regulate blood pressure and electrolyte balance, and produce hormones.
- **Kidney failure: When** the kidneys fail, waste accumulates in the body, which can be dangerous. Dialysis takes over to help eliminate this waste.

3. HOW DOES IT WORK?

- **Principle of diffusion: Blood** waste passes through a semi-permeable membrane into a solution (dialysate) which attracts it. The concentration of this waste is

higher in the blood than in the dialysate, hence the movement of the waste.
- **Osmotic balance:** The elimination of excess water from the blood is achieved by osmosis, where water moves from an area of low solute concentration to an area of high concentration.

4. TYPES OF DIALYSIS
- **Haemodialysis:** Blood is pumped from the body to a dialysis machine, which filters it and returns it to the body.
- **Peritoneal dialysis:** Dialysis fluid is introduced into the abdominal cavity through a catheter. Waste products are eliminated through the membrane of the peritoneum and the liquid is then drained.

5. IMPORTANCE OF DIALYSATE
- **Composition:** Dialysate is a specially formulated solution to help eliminate waste and balance electrolyte levels in the blood.
- **Role:** As well as eliminating waste, dialysate compensates for electrolyte imbalances (such as potassium or calcium) to maintain a healthy environment for the body.

Dialysis is a vital medical intervention for many people suffering from kidney failure. Although complex, its fundamental understanding relies on the principles of diffusion and osmosis to eliminate waste and balance substances in the blood. A basic knowledge of this procedure helps patients and their families to understand and manage this essential part of their medical treatment.

• Step-by-step procedure
Although each dialysis centre may have its own specific procedures, here is a general sequence of steps followed

during a dialysis session, focusing mainly on haemodialysis, the most common form.

1. PREPARING THE PATIENT
- **Clinical assessment:** Checking vital signs (blood pressure, pulse, temperature).
- **Weighing:** To determine the amount of water to be removed during the session.
- **Examination of the vascular access:** looking for signs of infection or dysfunction.

2. PREPARING THE DIALYSIS MACHINE
- **Cleaning:** Make sure the machine is clean and disinfected.
- **Dialysate setting:** According to the patient's specific needs.
- **Preparing the filter (dialyser):** Installation and priming with saline solution.
- **Testing the machine:** To make sure there are no leaks and that everything is working properly.

3. CONNECTING THE PATIENT TO THE MACHINE
- **Cleaning the access:** The access (fistula, graft or catheter) is cleaned with an antiseptic.
- **Insertion of needles:** In the case of fistulas or grafts, two needles are inserted: one to withdraw the blood (arterial needle) and the other to return it (venous needle).
- **Catheter connection:** If the patient has a catheter, it is connected directly to the machine's tubes.

4. INITIATION OF DIALYSIS
- **Starting the pump:** Blood begins to be pumped out of the body, passing through the dialyser where it is cleaned and then returned to the body.
- **Continuous monitoring:** Parameters such as blood pressure, heart rate and blood flow rate are monitored

regularly. Vital signs are generally taken every 30 minutes.

5. DURING DIALYSIS
- **Fluid removal:** The machine is set to remove a certain amount of fluid from the body, depending on the weight gained between treatments.
- **Symptom monitoring:** Look for signs of hypotension, cramps, headaches or other symptoms. Parameters can be adjusted if necessary.
- **Activities:** Some patients can read, watch television, sleep or even work on a computer during dialysis.

6. END OF DIALYSIS SESSION
- **Machine shutdown: Once the** session time has elapsed, the machine is shut down.
- **Removing the needles:** The needles are removed, and pressure is applied to prevent bleeding.
- **Post-dialysis weighing:** To determine the amount of fluid removed.
- **Post-dialysis assessment:** Check for any symptoms or complications and check vital signs.

7. DISCONNECTION AND FOLLOW-UP
- **Cleaning the access:** The access is cleaned and disinfected again.
- **Data recording:** All relevant information is recorded in the patient's medical file.
- **Instructions:** If necessary, instructions for the period between sessions are provided.

The dialysis procedure, although routine for medical staff and many patients, is a meticulous process requiring constant attention to detail to ensure the safety and effectiveness of the treatment. Understanding the steps involved can help patients and those around them to better understand what they are going through and to work more effectively with the medical team.

• Vascular access management

Vascular access is essential for haemodialysis. It is the site where blood is removed from the body and returned after being cleaned by the dialysis machine. Appropriate management of vascular access is crucial to ensuring effective and uncomplicated dialysis sessions.

1. TYPES OF VASCULAR ACCESS
- **Arteriovenous fistula (AVF):** Created surgically by connecting an artery to a vein, usually in the arm. It is the preferred access because of its longevity and low risk of infection.
- **Arteriovenous graft:** Uses a synthetic tube to connect an artery to a vein, usually when the patient's blood vessels are not suitable for creating an AVF.
- **Central venous catheter:** Inserted into a large vein, usually in the neck or chest. It is used when haemodialysis needs to be started quickly, but is not recommended as a long-term solution.

2. MONITORING VASCULAR ACCESS
- **Physical examination:** The access should be palpated and auscultated regularly to detect the "thrill" (vibration) and "noise" (buzzing) characteristic of good blood flow.
- **Monitoring complications:** looking for signs of infection, thrombosis, stenosis or aneurysm.
- **Flow tests:** Blood flow measurements to assess access performance.

3. MAINTENANCE AND CARE
- **Cleaning:** The access must be carefully cleaned before each dialysis session to reduce the risk of infection.

- **Protection:** Avoid wearing tight clothing, sleeping on access or using your arm to carry heavy loads.
- **Consideration of haematoma: In the** event of post-dialysis bleeding, adequate pressure should be applied. Any significant haematoma should be assessed by a healthcare professional.

4. COMPLICATION MANAGEMENT
- **Infections:** Signs of infection, such as redness, warmth, pain or discharge, must be treated immediately. Antibiotics may be necessary.
- **Thrombosis:** The presence of clots can block access. Treatments include thrombolysis or surgery.
- **Stenosis:** A narrowing of the access may require angioplasty or surgery to correct it.

5. REPLACEMENT OR CLOSURE OF ACCESS
- **Access failure:** If an access fails and cannot be repaired, a new access may be required.
- **Closure:** If a patient no longer requires dialysis (e.g. after a kidney transplant), the access can be left in place or surgically closed, depending on the circumstances.

Effective management of vascular accesses is essential to ensure that patients receive optimal dialysis treatment. The choice of access, its regular monitoring and the prevention of complications are key elements of this management. Open communication between the patient and the dialysis team is essential to identify problems early and ensure appropriate care.

Peritoneal dialysis

• Understanding peritoneal dialysis

Peritoneal dialysis is a form of treatment that uses the patient's peritoneal membrane as a filter to remove waste and excess fluid from the body. This membrane covers the abdomen and internal organs. Peritoneal dialysis offers an alternative to haemodialysis, the most commonly used type of dialysis.

1. HOW DOES IT WORK?

- **Dialysis solution:** A special solution, often called dialysate, is introduced into the abdominal cavity through a catheter. This solution draws waste products and excess fluid through the peritoneal membrane.
- **Exchange:** After a certain period of time, the dialysis solution is drained from the abdomen and replaced by a new one. This process is called exchange.

2. TYPES OF PERITONEAL DIALYSIS

- **Continuous ambulatory peritoneal dialysis (CAPD):** Exchanges are carried out manually, usually 4 times a day at regular intervals.
- **Automated peritoneal dialysis (APD):** A machine called a "cycler" carries out exchanges during the night while the patient is asleep.

3. BENEFITS

- **Flexibility:** Allows the patient a degree of mobility and can be carried out at home.
- **Fewer dietary restrictions:** Compared with haemodialysis.

- **Haemodynamic stability:** Fewer rapid fluctuations in blood pressure, which is gentler on the heart and blood vessels.

4. LIMITATIONS
- **Self-management requirement:** The patient must be able to make the exchanges themselves or have someone to help them.
- **Risk of infection:** In particular peritonitis, an infection of the peritoneal membrane.
- **Space requirements:** To store supplies at home.

5. CATHETER INSTALLATION
- **Minor surgery:** To insert a flexible catheter into the abdomen.
- **Waiting period:** The catheter is usually left in place for several weeks to heal before starting exchanges.

6. MONITORING AND FOLLOW-UP
- **Regular visits to the nephrologist:** To assess the effectiveness of treatment and monitor renal function.
- **Ongoing education:** To ensure that the patient understands how to perform exchanges correctly and how to recognise signs of infection or other complications.

7. POSSIBLE COMPLICATIONS
- **Peritonitis:** Infection of the peritoneal membrane, recognisable by abdominal pain, cloudy dialysate and fever.
- **Blockages or leaks:** From the catheter, which may require adjustments or interventions.
- **Hernias:** Due to the increase in abdominal pressure caused by the dialysate.

Peritoneal dialysis is a viable option for many patients with kidney failure. It offers greater independence and flexibility than haemodialysis, although it does require the active participation of the patient. As with any form of treatment, it is essential to be well informed, to have good communication with the medical team and to follow the instructions carefully in order to maximise the benefits and minimise the risks.

• Connection and disconnection techniques

Connection and disconnection are critical steps in the dialysis process, particularly for haemodialysis, which requires direct access to the patient's blood stream. It is crucial that these steps are carried out with precision and hygiene to prevent complications, particularly infections.

CONNECTION TO THE DIALYSIS MACHINE

1. Preparation :
   - **Checking the patient's identity:** Always confirm the patient's identity before starting.
   - **Preparing the area: Make sure** the work area is clean and well lit.
   - **Hand washing:** This is an essential step in preventing infection.
   - **Patient preparation:** Check the access point (arteriovenous fistula, graft or catheter).

2. Connection :
   - **Cleaning the access site:** Use an antiseptic solution to clean the access site.
   - **Needle insertion:** For AVF or grafting, insert the needles - one for the blood supply and one for the return.
   - **Connection to the circuit:** Connect the needles to the machine's dialysis circuit tubing.
   - **Starting the machine:** Follow the instructions on the machine to start dialysis.

DISCONNECTING THE DIALYSIS MACHINE

1. End of dialysis session:
   - **Stopping the machine:** Follow the instructions to stop the machine safely.
   - **Clamping the tubing:** Clamp the tubing to prevent any bleeding or air entering.
   - **Needle removal:** Carefully remove the needles from the access site.

2. Care after disconnection:
   - **Compression of the site:** Apply firm pressure with a sterile compress to the access site to prevent bleeding.
   - **Monitoring: Make** sure that the bleeding has stopped and that the site is clean. Apply a dressing if necessary.
   - **Waste management:** Dispose of used needles and other supplies in accordance with medical waste management guidelines.
   - **Hand washing:** Always wash your hands after finishing work.

Key points:
   - Sterility and cleanliness are essential to avoid complications.
   - Always follow the establishment's protocols and the machine's instructions.
   - Make sure the patient is comfortable and well informed throughout the process.
   - Monitor the patient during dialysis to detect any signs of complications or discomfort.

Connection and disconnection are delicate procedures which, when carried out correctly, can ensure a safe and effective dialysis session for the patient. It is essential to focus on safety, cleanliness and maintaining open communication with the patient throughout the procedure.

• Specific care and common problems

Providing care during dialysis sessions requires constant attention to detail and prevention. Many problems can arise during dialysis, and being prepared to identify and manage them is essential for the patient's well-being.

1. HYPOTENSION:

- **Cause:** Rapid withdrawal of too much fluid, reaction to dialysis solutions, or patient co-morbidities.
- **Symptoms:** Dizziness, nausea, blurred vision, fatigue.
- **Care:** Reduce the rate of fluid withdrawal, elevate the patient's legs, administer saline solutions if necessary.

2. MUSCLE CRAMPS:

- **Cause:** Rapid withdrawal of liquid, electrolyte imbalance.
- **Symptoms:** Sudden muscle pain, usually in the legs.
- **Care:** Reduce the rate of fluid withdrawal, gently stretch the affected muscle, adjust the electrolyte imbalance if necessary.

3. HEADACHES:

- **Cause:** Hypotension, electrolyte imbalance or hypertension.
- **Symptoms:** Persistent pain in the head, sometimes accompanied by nausea or sensitivity to light.
- **Care:** Adjust blood pressure, administer analgesics if necessary, monitor electrolyte levels.

4. NAUSEA AND VOMITING:

- **Cause:** Rapid withdrawal of fluid, electrolyte imbalance, medication, or reaction to dialysis solution.
- **Symptoms:** Stomach discomfort, vomiting.
- **Care:** Slow the rate of fluid withdrawal, administer anti-nausea medication, monitor electrolyte levels.

5. PRURITUS (ITCHING):
- **Cause:** Accumulation of waste products, calcium and phosphorus imbalance.
- **Symptoms:** Persistent itching, often worse during or after dialysis.
- **Care:** Moisturising the skin, adjusting calcium and phosphorus levels, antipruritic medication.

6. FEVER AND CHILLS:
- **Cause:** Infection, reaction to dialyser membrane or dialysis solution.
- **Symptoms:** High body temperature, chills, fatigue.
- **Care:** Identify and treat infection, monitor temperature, change dialyser membrane or solution if necessary.

7. VASCULAR ACCESS MALFUNCTION:
- **Cause:** Thrombosis, stenosis or infection.
- **Symptoms:** Low blood flow during dialysis, swelling, redness or tenderness around the access site.
- **Care:** Ultrasound assessment, anticoagulants, surgery if necessary.

8. HEART PROBLEMS:
- **Cause:** Fluid overload, hypertension, electrolyte imbalances.
- **Symptoms:** Shortness of breath, chest pain, palpitations.
- **Care:** Adjustment of fluid volume, cardiac medication, cardiac consultation.

Every patient is unique, and it is crucial to monitor each individual closely for symptoms and signs of complications during dialysis. Early and appropriate intervention can prevent more serious complications and ensure patient safety and comfort. Ongoing training and updating of knowledge is essential for all healthcare professionals working in a dialysis service.

Chapter 5:
THE DIALYSIS PATIENT

Psychological aspects dialysis

• Adapting to life on dialysis

Discovering that you need to start dialysis sessions can be a major upheaval for many patients. Adapting to this new reality takes time, understanding and constant support. This section provides an overview of the challenges faced by patients and strategies for overcoming them.

1. UNDERSTANDING DIALYSIS :

- **The importance of education:** The first step is to understand what dialysis is and why it is necessary.
- **How the machine works:** Having a basic understanding of the process can help reduce anxiety.

2. TIME MANAGEMENT :

- **Frequency of sessions:** Patients need to fit dialysis sessions into their schedule, often three times a week for haemodialysis.
- **Duration:** Each session lasts several hours, which can disrupt your daily routine.

3. DIETARY CHANGES :

- **Dietary restrictions:** Dialysis patients often have to watch their intake of fluids, potassium, phosphorus and salt.
- **Consultation with a dietician:** A professional can help you draw up a suitable eating plan.

4. EMOTIONAL ASPECTS :
- **Psychological support:** Dialysis can lead to feelings of sadness, frustration or anger.
- **Support groups:** Talking to others in a similar situation can offer perspective and support.

5. PHYSICAL ACTIVITY :
- **Appropriate exercise:** Although fatigue can be a side effect, moderate exercise can improve the feeling of well-being.
- **Consultation with a physiotherapist:** To establish a suitable exercise programme.

6. WORK AND LEISURE :
- **Work adjustments:** Inform your employer and discuss possible adjustments.
- **Travel:** Planning is essential for those who wish to travel. Dialysis centres are available in many regions, but sessions need to be arranged in advance.

7. SOCIAL AND FAMILY RELATIONS :
- **Communication:** Explain to family and friends what it means to be on dialysis and how they can help.
- **Participation in activities:** Finding ways to stay involved in social activities while taking dialysis needs into account.

8. FUTURE PROSPECTS :
- **Kidney transplant:** For some people, a kidney transplant is an option to consider.
- **Home dialysis:** With appropriate training, some patients opt for home dialysis for greater flexibility.

Adapting to life with dialysis requires major adjustments in many aspects of daily life. However, with the right support, information and a proactive attitude, patients can lead fulfilling lives while effectively managing their condition.

• Psychological and social support

The impact of dialysis on a patient's quality of life is significant. Not only does the treatment involve physical changes, but it also creates emotional and social challenges. Appropriate psychological and social support is therefore essential to help patients adapt to this new reality.

1. RECOGNISING EMOTIONAL CHALLENGES :
- **Common feelings:** Denial, anger, sadness, anxiety, depression, and frustration.
- **The stages of bereavement:** Understanding the stages of bereavement to better support patients.

2. MENTAL HEALTH PROFESSIONALS :
- **Psychologists:** Specialised in supporting patients with chronic illnesses.
- **Advisors:** Helps you manage the feelings and emotions associated with dialysis.

3. SUPPORT GROUPS :
- **Regular meetings:** Spaces where patients can share their experiences and support each other.
- **Online forums and communities:** A place to talk to other patients from all over the world.

4. SUPPORT FROM FAMILY AND FRIENDS :
- **Key role:** Relatives are often the first line of support.
- **Educating the family:** helping them to understand the dialysis process so that they can better support the patient.

5. ADAPTING TO THE NEW REALITY :
- **Recognising your limits:** Accepting life's new constraints.

- **Looking for new activities:** Finding hobbies to suit your new routine.

6. SOCIAL SUPPORT :
- **Social workers:** Can help identify and access local resources for patients.
- **Assistance programmes:** For financial needs, transport or home care.

7. INTEGRATION INTO THE WORKPLACE AND SOCIETY :
- **Work arrangements:** Discussions with the employer about flexible working hours or adaptations to the job.
- **Back to society:** How to deal with other people's perceptions and questions.

8. WORKSHOPS AND TRAINING :
- **Stress management:** relaxation techniques, meditation and breathing.
- **Therapeutic education:** Understanding your illness and treatments to live better with it.

9. FUTURE PROSPECTS :
- **Planning:** Consider the future, including the possibility of a transplant.
- **Living will:** Discussions on advance care directives.

Psychological and social support is a crucial pillar of care for dialysis patients. It is essential that carers recognise the importance of this aspect and provide or direct patients to appropriate resources. A holistic approach to care, taking into account both physical and emotional needs, will lead to a better quality of life for the patient.

Dietetics in dialysis

• Specific nutritional requirements

Nutrition plays an essential role in the overall well-being of dialysis patients. Due to the physiological changes associated with kidney disease, these patients may have specific nutritional needs that are crucial to understand and manage.

1. INTRODUCTION :

- **The importance of nutrition:** Why an appropriate diet is crucial for dialysis patients.

2. PROTEIN :

- **Increased needs:** Dialysis can lead to a loss of protein, thus increasing needs.
- **Sources of protein:** Meat, fish, eggs, dairy products, pulses.

3. ELECTROLYTES :

- Potassium :
    - Restrictions often necessary.
    - High content foods: bananas, oranges, potatoes, spinach.
    - Low-content foods: apples, grapes, strawberries, cucumbers.
- Phosphorus :
    - Reduction often recommended.
    - Foods to avoid: dairy products, nuts, beans, cereals.
    - Use of phosphorus binders.
- Sodium :
    - Control intake to manage blood pressure and fluid volume.
    - Avoid processed foods and commercial sauces.

4. FLUIDS :

- **Limitations:** Depending on residual urine production and type of dialysis.
- **Weight monitoring:** A way of assessing fluid balance.

5. CALORIES :

- **Energy requirements:** May vary according to activity level and body weight.
- **Energy sources:** Complex carbohydrates, healthy fats, proteins.

6. VITAMINS AND MINERALS :

- **Vitamin D:** Often required as a supplement due to altered metabolism.
- **Iron:** Important for preventing or treating anaemia associated with kidney disease.
- **Folic acid and vitamin B12:** For healthy red blood cells.

7. SUPPLEMENTS AND MEDICINES :

- **Necessity:** When and why they are prescribed.
- **Interactions: It** is important to contact your doctor and pharmacist.

8. FOODS TO AVOID :

- **Preservatives and additives :** May contain elements that are harmful to the kidneys.
- **Processed foods:** Often rich in sodium, phosphorus and potassium.

9. PRACTICAL ADVICE :

- **Meal planning:** Preparing balanced meals, taking restrictions into account.
- **Reading labels:** To monitor sodium, potassium and phosphorus intakes.

10. WORKING WITH A DIETICIAN :
- **Role of the dietician:** Personalising meal plans, education and monitoring.
- **Regular consultations:** Importance of updates and adjustments based on clinical developments.

Adapting dietary habits is essential to optimising the health and quality of life of dialysis patients. A collaborative approach with healthcare professionals, in particular dieticians specialising in nephrology, ensures that specific nutritional needs are met.

• Practical advice for a suitable diet
A balanced and appropriate diet is essential for dialysis patients to prevent complications and improve their quality of life. Here is some practical advice to help patients make the best possible dietary choices while respecting their specific needs.

1. PLAN YOUR MEALS:
- **Plan ahead:** Plan your weekly menus to ensure a balanced diet.
- **Shopping list:** Prepare a list before you go shopping to avoid unnecessary temptations.

2. COOK AT HOME :
- **Total control:** You know exactly which ingredients are used.
- **Explore new recipes:** Discover diet-friendly yet delicious dishes.

3. USE HERBS AND SPICES:
- **Alternative to salt:** Season your dishes with fresh or dried herbs to reduce your sodium intake.
- **Reading labels:** Some commercial spice blends may contain sodium.

4. LIMIT PROCESSED FOODS:

- **High sodium and phosphorus content:** Industrial foods are often rich in additives and preservatives.
- **Opt for fresh food:** Choose fresh, unprocessed food for better nutritional control.

5. BE CAREFUL WITH DRINKS:

- **Fluid monitoring:** Keep track of your daily fluid intake.
- **Avoid soft drinks:** especially those rich in phosphates.
- **Choose water, herbal teas** and other additive-free drinks.

6. OPT FOR QUALITY PROTEIN SOURCES:

- **Variety:** Alternate between meat, fish, eggs and dairy products (depending on your doctor's recommendations).
- **Avoid processed meats:** such as sausages and cold meats, which often contain a lot of salt.

7. BE CAREFUL WITH FRUIT AND VEGETABLES:

- **Potassium:** Some fruit and vegetables are very rich in potassium. Learn to identify them and eat them in the right quantities.
- **Cooking techniques:** Boiling can help reduce the potassium content of certain vegetables.

8. CHOOSE LOW-PHOSPHORUS DAIRY PRODUCTS:

- **Choice:** Almond or rice milk can be an alternative to cow's milk.
- **Cheeses:** Some cheeses contain more phosphorus than others. Find out more.

9. KEEP AN EYE ON THE DESSERTS:

- **Sugar:** Limit your intake of sugar and very sweet desserts.

- **Healthy choices:** Opt for fresh fruit or homemade desserts with a reduced sugar content.

10. INFORM AND EDUCATE YOURSELF:
- **Meetings with a dietician:** A professional can help you understand and adapt your diet.
- **Reading:** Get hold of specialist books or online resources to help you make informed food choices.

The right diet is essential for dialysis patients. By following a few rules and being vigilant, it is possible to enjoy a delicious diet while meeting the specific needs associated with kidney disease. The key is to be well informed, listen to your body, and work closely with your healthcare professionals.

Life beyond the dialysis centre

• Social and professional integration
The social and professional integration of dialysis patients is a major factor in their quality of life. Living with dialysis often means juggling sessions, symptoms, dietary constraints and medical appointments while trying to lead a "normal" life. Here's a look at how integration can be promoted and the challenges these patients face.

1. INTRODUCTION :
- **Importance of integration: This is why it is** essential to maintain a social and professional life despite dialysis.

2. PROFESSIONAL CHALLENGES :
- **Adjustments to working hours:** Need to adjust working hours around dialysis sessions.

- **Fatigue:** How to manage post-dialysis fatigue at work.
- **Discrimination:** Overcoming prejudice and stigma in the workplace.

3. SUPPORT IN THE WORKPLACE :
- **Communication with the employer:** Transparency and awareness-raising are essential.
- **Reasonable accommodation:** such as extra breaks or a space to rest.
- **Colleague training:** Raising awareness of kidney disease and dialysis.

4. SOCIAL LIFE AND DIALYSIS :
- **Planning:** Organising social activities around the dialysis schedule.
- **Acceptance:** Understanding that some days will be better than others.
- **Travel:** How to travel while on dialysis.

5. EMOTIONAL SUPPORT :
- **Support groups:** sharing experiences with other people in the same situation.
- **Therapy:** Working with a professional to manage stress and anxiety.
- **Family and friends:** Draw on a support network.

6. ADAPTED ACTIVITIES :
- **Gentle sports:** such as walking, yoga or swimming.
- **Hobbies:** Find activities that aren't physically demanding but are rewarding.

7. CONTINUING EDUCATION :
- **Adapted programmes:** Schools or universities offering flexible timetables.

- **Online courses:** An option for those who find it difficult to attend face-to-face courses.

8. RETURNING TO WORK AFTER A BREAK :
- **Preparation:** Feeling physically and emotionally ready.
- **Job search:** Find a job that can adapt to the needs of dialysis patients.

9. THE IMPORTANCE OF AUTONOMY :
- **Learn to dialyse at home:** This option can offer greater flexibility.
- **Taking charge of your health:** knowing your needs and limits.

Social and professional integration is key to the well-being of dialysis patients. While there can be challenges, with the right support, communication and some adaptation, it is possible to lead a fulfilling and productive life while managing the demands of dialysis.

• Physical activities and leisure
Physical activity and leisure are essential for everyone, including those on dialysis. They contribute not only to physical health, but also to emotional and mental balance. For dialysis patients, engaging in suitable activities can improve quality of life, boost self-esteem and help manage the stress associated with their medical condition.

1. INTRODUCTION :
- **Benefits of physical activity:** The importance of staying active for heart health, endurance and muscle strength.
- **Impact on emotional well-being:** How physical activity can improve mood, reduce stress and promote a sense of achievement.

2. SELECT A SUITABLE ACTIVITY :
- **Personal assessment:** Understanding your limits and listening to your body.
- **Medical consultation:** Talk to your nephrologist or GP before starting any new activity.

3. RECOMMENDED PHYSICAL ACTIVITIES :
- **Walking:** An excellent starting point for almost everyone.
- **Swimming:** Low impact on the joints while providing a full-body workout.
- **Cycling:** Whether on a stationary bike or in the open air, this is an excellent way to strengthen your legs.
- **Yoga:** Improves flexibility and strength and offers mental relaxation.
- **Strengthening exercises:** Use of light weights or elastic bands.

4. MAKE PHYSICAL ACTIVITY PART OF YOUR DAILY ROUTINE :
- **Stretching:** Light stretching in the morning or before dialysis sessions.
- **Short walks:** Incorporate short walks throughout the day.
- **Incorporating exercise during dialysis:** Certain movements can be performed even during dialysis.

5. ADAPTED LEISURE ACTIVITIES :
- **Gardening: A** soothing activity that also provides physical exercise.
- **Arts and crafts:** Painting, knitting, pottery to stimulate the mind while offering relaxation.
- **Music:** Learning an instrument or simply listening to music to relax.
- **Board games and puzzles:** A way of socialising and stimulating the mind.

6. THE IMPORTANCE OF SOCIALISATION :
- **Join a group:** walking groups, swimming or yoga clubs to connect with others.
- **Group activities:** Engage in activities that allow you to socialise and share experiences.

7. SAFETY ADVICE :
- **Hydration:** Drink enough water, bearing in mind the restrictions associated with dialysis.
- **Appropriate equipment:** Wear suitable footwear and clothing.
- **Listen to your body:** Recognise when to take a break or when to stop an activity.

8. OVERCOMING CHALLENGES:
- **Managing fatigue:** how to adapt physical activity when you feel tired or after a dialysis session.
- **Avoid overdoing it:** Strike a balance between staying active and not overdoing it.

Staying active and engaging in leisure activities is beneficial on several levels for dialysis patients. Not only does it help physically, but it also plays a crucial role in mental and emotional well-being. The key is to choose suitable activities, consult healthcare professionals regularly and listen to yourself so that you can make the most of every moment.

Chapter 6:
DEVELOPMENTS AND OUTLOOK

The latest innovations in dialysis

Dialysis, like other medical fields, has benefited from major technological advances and research in recent years. These innovations aim to improve patients' quality of life, increase the effectiveness of treatment and reduce potential complications. Here's a look at some of the most significant innovations in dialysis up to my last update point in 2021.

1. INTRODUCTION :
- **The evolution of dialysis:** A brief history of how dialysis has progressed over the decades.

2. PORTABLE DIALYSIS MACHINES :
- **Compact design: for** easy transport and dialysis on the move.
- **Benefits for the patient:** Greater flexibility and independence.

3. TELEMEDICINE IN DIALYSIS :
- **Remote monitoring:** healthcare professionals can monitor patients' dialysis sessions remotely.
- **Virtual consultations:** Patients can consult their nephrologist without having to travel in person.

4. IMPROVEMENTS IN DIALYSERS :
- **Increased efficiency:** Increased capacity to eliminate waste.
- **Biological compatibility:** Reduction in allergic reactions or complications.

5. NEEDLE-FREE DIALYSIS :

- **Technology under development:** Research to eliminate the need for needles during the dialysis process.
- **Potential benefits:** Less pain and risk of infection.

6. BIOARTIFICIAL IMPLANTS :

- **Bioartificial kidneys:** Devices combining living cells and synthetic elements to mimic kidney function.
- **Current progress:** How far has research progressed and what are the challenges ahead?

7. INNOVATION IN PERITONEAL DIALYSIS :

- **Dialysis solutions:** Improvements to increase efficiency and reduce irritation.
- **Automated systems:** Machines that regulate the filling, residence time and emptying processes.

8. WEARABLES AND SURVEILLANCE TECHNOLOGY :

- **Real-time monitoring devices:** Enable patients and doctors to track toxin levels and other indicators.
- **Intelligent alerts:** Notifications sent in the event of anomalies.

9. RESEARCH IN PROGRESS :

- **Tissue research:** Potential for creating more durable vascular accessories.
- **Regenerative dialysis:** Use of regenerative medicine to repair or replace failing kidney functions.

Innovations in dialysis bring hope to the millions of people around the world who depend on this technology for their survival. As research continues, the future looks bright for further improvements in the effectiveness of treatment and quality of life for patients.

Note: It is crucial to stress that research and innovation continue to evolve after 2021. Readers interested in the most recent advances should consult current sources of information in the medical field.

Renal transplantation

• When and why consider a transplant?
Kidney transplantation is a treatment option for many patients with advanced chronic kidney disease (CKD). The aim is to replace the function of failing kidneys with a kidney from a donor. This procedure can offer a better quality of life and a longer lifespan than dialysis, but it also involves challenges and risks.

1. INTRODUCTION :
- **Definition of a kidney transplant: What** is a transplant and how does it work?

2. ADVANTAGES OF TRANSPLANTATION OVER DIALYSIS :
- **Lifespan:** Transplant patients generally live longer than those on dialysis.
- **Quality of life:** Better energy, fewer dietary restrictions, less frequent medical treatment.
- **Economic costs:** In the long term, transplantation may be less expensive than dialysis.

3. WHEN TO CONSIDER TRANSPLANTATION :
- **Advanced stage of CKD:** Usually when the glomerular filtration rate (GFR) falls below 20 ml/min.
- **Before starting dialysis:** In some cases, a pre-emptive transplant is possible even before starting dialysis.
- **Age and general health:** Although age is not a strict contraindication, overall health is crucial.

4. SOURCES OF KIDNEYS FOR TRANSPLANTATION :

- **Living donors:** Usually family members, friends or sometimes altruistic donors.
- **Deceased donors:** People who have donated their organs after their death.

5. EVALUATION FOR TRANSPLANTATION :

- **Medical examination:** To determine physical suitability for transplantation.
- **Psychosocial assessment:** To examine the patient's ability to manage the demands of post-transplantation.
- **Compatibility:** Tests to determine the compatibility of the donor and recipient.

6. RISKS ASSOCIATED WITH TRANSPLANTATION :

- **Rejection:** The recipient's immune system may attack the new kidney.
- **Infections:** Immunosuppressive drugs can increase the risk of infections.
- **Side effects of medication:** The drugs required post-transplant may have side effects.
- **Recurrent diseases :** Certain kidney diseases may recur in the transplanted kidney.

7. LIFE AFTER A TRANSPLANT :

- **Regular medical monitoring:** Necessary to monitor the function of the new kidney.
- **Lifetime medication:** Immunosuppressive drugs are generally required for life.
- **Rehabilitation:** Return to a normal life with adaptations.

Kidney transplantation is an intervention that can offer a better quality of life to many patients with advanced CKD. However, it is a major decision that requires careful evaluation of the benefits and risks. Patients and their families must be well informed and involved in the decision-making process.

• The role of the nurse in preparing for transplantation

Preparing for a kidney transplant is a complex process that requires multidisciplinary coordination. The nurse plays a central role in this process, as the main person involved with the patient, providing education, preparation and emotional support. Let's take a closer look at the nurse's responsibilities during this crucial phase.

1. INTRODUCTION :

- **The importance of preparation:** Why adequate preparation is essential for successful transplantation.

2. PATIENT EDUCATION :

- **Transplant process:** Explain the different stages, from pre-operative assessments to surgery and post-operative care.
- **Risks and benefits:** Present the potential benefits and possible complications.
- **Medication:** Information on immunosuppressive drugs and their side effects.
- **Post-transplant lifestyle:** Discuss the lifestyle changes required after transplantation.

3. PRE-TRANSPLANT ASSESSMENT :

- **Coordination of tests:** Ensure that all necessary tests are carried out.
- **Interpreting results:** Helping the patient to understand the test results and their implications.
- **Vaccination monitoring:** Ensure that the patient is up to date with the vaccinations recommended prior to transplantation.

4. PSYCHOLOGICAL PREPARATION :
- **Assessment of emotional well-being:** Identify any concerns or fears the patient may have.
- **Emotional support:** providing empathetic listening and referring to additional resources if necessary (psychologists, support groups).

5. WORKING WITH THE MULTIDISCIPLINARY TEAM :
- **Care coordination:** working closely with nephrologists, surgeons, dieticians, social workers, etc.
- **Team meetings:** Attend meetings to discuss the patient's progress and any obstacles to transplantation.

6. PREPARING FOR THE DAY OF SURGERY :
- **Pre-operative checklist:** Ensure that all the necessary steps have been completed before the operation.
- **Fasting and medication:** Give instructions on dietary restrictions and taking medication before surgery.

7. PREPARING FOR THE TRIP :
- **Home care:** Educating patients and their families about post-operative care at home.
- **Warning signs:** Educate people about the signs of complications or rejection to watch out for.

8. ROLE IN POST-TRANSPLANT FOLLOW-UP :
- **Regular consultations:** Planning and carrying out patient follow-up after surgery.
- **Medication management:** Monitor medication adherence and adjust doses if necessary.

The nurse is a central pillar in the preparation for transplantation. As the main link between the patient and the medical team, their role is crucial in ensuring that the patient is well informed, prepared and supported throughout the process. Careful preparation can greatly influence the success of the transplant and the patient's overall well-being.

Ethical considerations on dialysis

Dialysis, as a vital treatment for many people suffering from kidney failure, raises a number of ethical issues. The dilemma between prolonging life and quality of life, fair access to treatment and end-of-life decisions are all issues that require in-depth ethical reflection.

1. INTRODUCTION :
- **Dialysis in context:** Presentation of dialysis as an essential but complex treatment.

2. LONGER LIFE VS. QUALITY OF LIFE :
- **The benefits of dialysis:** The ability of dialysis to prolong patients' lives.
- **The challenges of dialysis:** constraints, complications and the impact on patients' daily lives.
- **Ethical dilemmas:** How do you balance the desire to prolong life with the potential for suffering or reduced quality of life?

3. EQUITABLE ACCESS TO TREATMENT :
- **Disparities in access:** Not all patients have equal access to dialysis, depending on their geographical location, socio-economic situation, etc.
- **Prioritising patients:** How do you determine who receives treatment when resources are limited?
- **Cost of dialysis:** the ethical implications of meeting the costs of treatment.

4. END OF LIFE AND CESSATION OF DIALYSIS :

- **Respect for patient autonomy:** The patient's right to choose to stop dialysis.
- **Shared decision-making :** How can healthcare professionals help patients make an informed decision?
- **Religious and cultural considerations:** How do personal beliefs influence end-of-life decisions?

5. INFORMED CONSENT :

- **Full information:** Ensuring that patients fully understand the risks, benefits and alternatives.
- **Autonomous decision-making:** Respecting the patient's choices while ensuring that they are based on a clear understanding.

6. DIALYSIS IN CHILDREN AND THE ELDERLY :

- **Consent :** The ethical challenges of obtaining consent from minors and the elderly.
- **Prioritisation:** How can access to dialysis for these vulnerable groups be determined?
- **Quality of life:** The particular implications of dialysis for these populations.

7. INNOVATION AND RESEARCH :

- **Clinical trials:** the ethical dilemmas of patient participation in dialysis research.
- **New treatments :** How do you balance the hope of new treatments with the potential risks?

The ethical issues surrounding dialysis are complex and require careful consideration. As medicine continues to advance, healthcare professionals, patients and society as a whole must work together to address these challenges with compassion, respect and integrity.

Chapter 7:
RESOURCES AND TOOLS

Documentation tools for nurses

Documentation plays a crucial role in nursing care. Not only does it guarantee continuity of care, it also serves as a means of communication between healthcare professionals and provides a legal record of the care provided. Here is a list of essential documentation tools for nurses:

1. ELECTRONIC MEDICAL RECORDS (EMR) :
- **Overview:** Introduction to EMRs and their importance in the modern healthcare context.
- **Features:** Capability to enter, store, retrieve and share patient information.
- **Benefits:** Rapid access, fewer errors, improved coordination of care.

2. NURSING CARE RECORDS :
- **Care plans:** Drawing up, updating and monitoring individual care plans.
- **Progress notes:** Documentation of changes in the patient's condition and the interventions carried out.

3. SORTING TOOLS :
- **Pain scales:** Tools for assessing and documenting patient pain.
- **Assessment checklists:** Lists used to quickly assess a patient's condition on admission, during changes in condition or on discharge.

4. MOBILE APPLICATIONS FOR NURSES :
- **Medication guides:** Applications offering detailed information on medicines, their interactions, dosages, etc.
- **Medical calculators:** For drug dosages, body indices, conversions, etc.
- **Logbook:** Keep track of schedules, tasks and personal notes.

5. SPECIALISED REGISTERS :
- **Vaccination registers:** Tracking of vaccinations given and to be given.
- **Wound registers:** Documentation of wound care, including size, depth, appearance, etc.

6. ORDER MANAGEMENT SYSTEMS :
- **Electronic prescriptions:** to send, track and confirm medical prescriptions.
- **Diagnostic test orders:** Tools for requesting, tracking and receiving test results.

7. TRAINING AND ONLINE RESOURCES :
- **E-learning platforms:** Courses and training for continuing professional development.
- **Medical databases:** access to articles, studies and best practice guides.

8. COMMUNICATION TOOLS :
- **Secure electronic messaging systems:** For secure communication with other healthcare professionals.
- **Videoconferencing software:** For remote consultations or communication with specialists.

9. PATIENT MONITORING SYSTEMS :
- **Portable monitors:** To monitor patients' vital signs in real time.

- **Alert systems:** To signal any major change in a patient's condition.

With the rapid evolution of medical technology, it is crucial that nurses have the tools they need to effectively document their work, guarantee patient safety and improve the quality of care. Familiarity with and regular training in these tools are essential to keep up to date and optimise the delivery of care.

Associations and organisations for professional support

Nurses, like other healthcare professionals, benefit from the support and resources provided by various associations and organisations. These entities play an essential role in providing continuing education, networking opportunities, professional advocacy and support for specific issues or concerns. The following is a non-exhaustive list of notable associations and organizations for the professional support of nurses:

1. INTERNATIONAL ORGANISATIONS :
- **International Council of Nurses (ICN):** A federation of over 130 national nursing associations, representing the millions of nurses worldwide.

2. NATIONAL ASSOCIATIONS :
(This is based on a French-speaking context, but many regions will have similar equivalents)
- **Ordre National des Infirmiers (France):** Professional body regulating the nursing profession in France.
- **Canadian Nurses Association (CNA):** National professional organization for Canadian nurses.
- **Association Belge des Praticiens de l'Art Infirmier (ABP):** Represents nurses in Belgium.

- Fédération Suisse des Associations d'Infirmières et Infirmiers (FSAS): Represents nurses in Switzerland.

3. SPECIALIST ORGANISATIONS :
- French Association of Dialysis, Transplantation and Nephrology Nurses (AFIDTN) : For nurses specialising in nephrology.
- Association des Infirmières et Infirmiers en Urgence du Québec (AIIUQ): For nurses working in the emergency sector.
- French Society of Nurse Anaesthetists (SFIA): For nurse anaesthetists.

4. RESEARCH AND EDUCATION ASSOCIATIONS :
- Association pour le Développement de la Recherche en Soins Infirmiers (ADRSI): Promotes nursing research.
- **Institut de Formation en Soins Infirmiers (IFSI):** Organisations providing initial training for nurses.

5. SUPPORT AND WELFARE ORGANISATIONS :
- **Nightingale Trust:** Organisation dedicated to the well-being and support of nurses in times of stress or professional difficulty.
- **Support programmes for healthcare professionals**: Available in many regions, these programmes offer psychological support and resources to healthcare professionals.

6. NETWORKING GROUPS AND ONLINE FORUMS :
- **Infirmiers.com:** Information portal and forum for French-speaking nurses.
- **LinkedIn Groups specific to nurses:** Spaces to share resources, discuss professional issues and network with colleagues.

Membership or participation in these associations and organisations can greatly benefit nurses, whether they are at the start of their career or have years of experience. These structures provide a platform for continuing education, advocacy, professional support and personal growth. Nurses are advised to explore the options available in their region or specialty to maximise the benefits of these professional resources.

Advice on continuing training

Continuing education is essential for healthcare professionals, particularly nurses. Not only does it enable them to keep up to date with the latest medical advances, it also helps them to reinforce existing skills and acquire new ones. Here are some tips for effective and rewarding continuing education:

1. ASSESS YOUR NEEDS AND INTERESTS :
- Identify the areas in which you feel you might need more training, or those that you are particularly passionate about.

2. PLAN AHEAD:
- Make a note of the dates of any training courses, seminars or workshops you would like to attend.
- Plan your budget for training costs, travel, etc.

3. MAKE THE MOST OF ONLINE RESOURCES :
- Online courses (MOOCs), webinars and instructional videos can be effective and flexible ways of learning.
- Platforms such as Coursera, Udemy, and Khan Academy offer many relevant courses for healthcare professionals.

4. JOIN PROFESSIONAL ASSOCIATIONS:
- These organisations often offer continuing education courses, seminars and conferences at reduced rates for their members.
- They can also provide training credits or certifications.

5. READ REGULARLY :
- Subscribe to professional journals, newsletters or specialist blogs to keep up to date with the latest research and methods.

6. TAKE PART IN CONFERENCES AND WORKSHOPS:
- These events are not only educational, but also provide opportunities to network with colleagues and experts in the field.

7. LOOK FOR TRAINING OPPORTUNITIES IN YOUR WORKPLACE:
- Some healthcare establishments offer continuing education courses or sponsor participation in educational events.

8. GROUP TRAINING :
- Organise training sessions with colleagues. Collaborative learning can be more interactive and stimulating.

9. DON'T BE AFRAID TO STEP OUT OF YOUR COMFORT ZONE:
- Exploring areas of training not directly related to your specialism can enrich your professional outlook.

10. KEEP A RECORD OF YOUR TRAINING :
- Document all your continuing education activities. This can be useful for professional assessments, recognition or licence renewals.

11. ASK FOR FEEDBACK :

- After applying new knowledge or skills in your practice, ask for feedback from your colleagues or superiors to ensure that you are using them effectively.

12. BE CURIOUS:

- Medicine and nursing are constantly evolving. Cultivate a lifelong learning attitude by always being curious about new advances and techniques.

Continuing education is an investment in your career and in the quality of care you provide to your patients. By taking the initiative to continue your education and using the resources available to you, you can not only strengthen your professional skills, but also raise the standard of care in your field.

CONCLUSION

The journey of the dialysis nurse

The journey of each dialysis nurse is unique, shaped by personal experiences, encounters with patients, and the constant evolution of knowledge and skills. This journey often begins with a simple curiosity about a specialist area and develops into an exciting and rewarding career. This chapter explores that journey, from initial discovery to mastery of the specialty.

1. DISCOVERY: THE FIRST STEPS TOWARDS DIALYSIS
- **The first spark:** How a nurse discovers dialysis and what attracts him to the field.
- **Initial training:** The specific studies and training required to become a dialysis nurse.
- **First experiences:** The reality of working in dialysis, the challenges and rewards.

2. THE FIRST FEW YEARS: FAMILIARISING YOURSELF WITH THE SPECIALITY
- **Adapting to the environment:** The routine of a dialysis unit, the technology and the patients.
- **Building skills:** The importance of continuous training and learning on the job.
- **The first challenges:** managing complications, emergencies and the emotional aspect of managing chronic patients.

3. MASTERY: BECOMING A DIALYSIS EXPERT
- **Extending your knowledge:** Research, attending conferences and training other professionals.

- **The patient-nurse relationship:** Cultivating lasting relationships with patients and their families.
- **Innovation and leadership:** Taking initiatives to improve the care and operation of the dialysis unit.

4. UPS AND DOWNS: MANAGING EMOTIONAL CHALLENGES

- **Difficult times:** dealing with the loss of a patient, serious complications and stress.
- **Gratifying moments:** Celebrating successes, such as a successful transplant or an improvement in a patient's quality of life.
- **Finding balance:** The importance of taking care of yourself, finding sources of support and renewing your passion for your profession.

5. LOOKING TO THE FUTURE : DEVELOPMENTS AND ASPIRATIONS

- **Dialysis of the future:** Technological innovations and medical advances to come.
- **Broaden your horizons:** Explore other related fields, such as transplantation or research.
- **The legacy of a dialysis nurse:** The lasting impact left on patients, colleagues and the profession.

The journey of the dialysis nurse is one of learning, challenge, success and evolution. By recognising and valuing each stage of this journey, we can better understand the profound impact these professionals have on the lives of their patients and on the world of healthcare. This journey is a testament to dedication, expertise and compassion.

The importance of empathy and understanding

In the world of medicine, technical skill is paramount, but without empathy and understanding, the quality of care provided can be compromised. These human qualities are essential to establishing an effective therapeutic relationship with patients. In this chapter, we explore why empathy and understanding are crucial for any healthcare professional, particularly those working in specialist areas such as dialysis.

1. DEFINITIONS: EMPATHY VS. SYMPATHY
- **Understanding empathy:** Putting yourself in the other person's shoes without judgement.
- **The difference with sympathy:** feeling for the other vs. feeling with the other.

2. EMPATHY AS A THERAPEUTIC TOOL
- **Establishing a connection:** How empathy facilitates a relationship of trust with the patient.
- **Improving compliance:** The importance of good communication to encourage patients to follow treatment and advice.

3. THE BENEFITS OF EMPATHY FOR HEALTHCARE PROFESSIONALS
- **Reducing burn-out:** How an empathic approach can help manage work-related stress.
- **Improved job satisfaction:** The pleasure of providing patient-centred care.

4. THE CHALLENGES OF EMPATHY IN PRACTICE
- **Avoid emotional overload:** Strike a balance between getting emotionally involved and maintaining a professional distance.

- **The limits of empathy:** Recognising when to step back or ask for support.

5. UNDERSTANDING: BEYOND EMPATHY
- **Knowing the patient as an individual: taking into account the patient**'s personal history, beliefs and concerns.
- **Cultural aspects:** Understanding and respecting cultural differences in order to provide appropriate care.

6. CULTIVATING EMPATHY AND UNDERSTANDING: ADVICE FOR PROFESSIONALS
- **Further training:** Courses and workshops on empathic communication.
- **Peer supervision and support:** Discussing experiences and challenges with colleagues.
- **Mindfulness practices:** Techniques for remaining centred and present for each patient.

Empathy and understanding are not simply "soft skills"; they are essential to providing quality care. They enable us to see the patient as a whole, going beyond a simple medical diagnosis to consider the human being with his or her emotions, concerns and hopes. By practising empathy and understanding, healthcare professionals can not only improve the quality of care, but also find a deeper meaning in their work.

Towards a future full of hope and progress

At a time when medicine is evolving at breakneck speed, dialysis, too, is witnessing promising innovations. Technological advances, combined with a better understanding of patients' needs, are paving the way for a future in which people suffering from kidney failure can lead even more normal and fulfilling lives.

1. THE CURRENT DIALYSIS LANDSCAPE
- **The limitations of current technologies:** An overview of the challenges facing patients and carers.
- **The impact on quality of life:** How current dialysis affects patients' daily lives.

2. TECHNOLOGICAL INNOVATIONS IN DIALYSIS
- **Portable machines:** Lighter, more compact devices for dialysis at home or on the move.
- **Biotechnology:** artificial kidneys and the hope they represent for less invasive treatment.
- **Telemedicine:** remote patient monitoring for early intervention in the event of complications.

3. MORE PERSONALISED TREATMENTS
- **Precision medicine:** how genetics and data analysis can help tailor treatments.
- **Adapted protocols:** Care designed around the individual rather than a standard.

4. PREVENTION AS THE KEYSTONE
- **Patient education: Raising** awareness of the causes and prevention of kidney failure.
- **Screening programmes:** Identifying people at risk for early intervention.

5. THE ROLE OF EMPATHY AND UNDERSTANDING IN THIS FUTURE
- **More holistic care:** combining technology and humanity to provide better care.
- **The importance of listening:** understanding patients' aspirations and concerns in this new medical landscape.

6. WORKING TOGETHER FOR A BETTER FUTURE

- **The importance of partnerships:** collaboration between researchers, doctors, patients and companies.
- **The Power of Community:** How patients and carers can unite to influence health policy and research.

The future of dialysis, with its innovations and improvements, is a source of hope for many people around the world. By placing patients' needs and aspirations at the heart of these advances, we are moving towards a time when kidney failure will no longer be a sentence to a limited life, but rather one of many medical challenges, with advanced and appropriate solutions. Hope and progress, hand in hand, light the way towards a better future for all.

GLOSSARY OF MEDICAL TERMS

A
- **Anemia:** Reduction in the number of red blood cells in the blood, which can lead to tiredness and paleness.
- **Anticoagulant : A** drug that prevents the coagulation (thickening) of blood.
- **Artery:** Blood vessel that carries blood from the heart to the rest of the body.

B
- **Biopsy:** removal of a small sample of tissue for microscopic examination.
- **Renal check-up:** series of tests to assess the function of the kidneys.

C
- **Catheter:** flexible tube inserted into a vein or another part of the body to administer medicines, draw blood or carry out other procedures.
- **Creatinine:** Chemical substance filtered by the kidneys, often measured to assess renal function.

D
- **Dialysate:** Solution used in dialysis to eliminate blood waste.
- **Dialyzer:** Device used to filter blood during dialysis.

E
- **Electrolyte:** Chemical substance, such as sodium or potassium, which is essential for the body's vital functions.

- **Erythropoietin (EPO):** Hormone produced by the kidneys which stimulates the production of red blood cells.

F

- **Filtration:** Process by which the kidneys eliminate waste products from the blood.

G

- **Glomerulus:** Small structure in the kidneys where blood filtration takes place.

H

- **Haemodialysis: A** type of dialysis that uses a machine to filter waste from the blood.
- **Hypertension:** Increase in blood pressure.

I

- **Renal insufficiency:** Inability of the kidneys to filter blood properly.

J

K

- **Kalemia:** concentration of potassium in the blood.

L

M

- **Metabolite:** Chemical by-product of cellular activity, often filtered by the kidneys.

N

- **Nephrology:** Branch of medicine specialising in kidney diseases.
- **Nephron:** Functional unit of the kidneys, comprising the glomerulus and the tubules.

O

P

- **Peritoneum:** Membrane lining the abdominal cavity and enveloping the organs, used in peritoneal dialysis.
- **Proteinuria:** Presence of protein in the urine, a potential sign of kidney problems.

Q

R

- **Kidney:** Organ responsible for filtering blood and producing urine.

S

- **Sodium:** Essential electrolyte for fluid balance and other body functions.

T

- **Toxin:** Harmful substance that can accumulate in the blood if the kidneys are not working properly.

U

- **Urea:** Waste produced by protein metabolism and filtered by the kidneys.
- **Urologist:** Doctor specialising in diseases of the urinary tract and male reproductive system.

V

- **Vein:** Blood vessel that transports blood from organs and tissues to the heart.

W

X

Y

Z

Please note that this glossary is simplified and intended for a non-specialist audience. For a more detailed version, specialist medical sources should be consulted.

REFERENCES AND RECOMMENDED READING

1. General works on nephrology
   - *Brenner & Rector's The Kidney.* Taal MW, Chertow GM, Marsden PA, Skorecki K, Yu ASL, Brenner BM (eds). Elsevier.
   - *Comprehensive Clinical Nephrology.* Feehally J, Floege J, Johnson RJ, Tonelli M (eds). Elsevier.

2. Specialisation in dialysis
   - *Handbook of Dialysis.* Daugirdas JT, Blake PG, Ing TS (eds). Wolters Kluwer.
   - *Clinical Dialysis.* Nissenson AR, Fine RN (eds). McGraw-Hill Education.

3. Nephrology nursing care
   - *Renal Nursing.* Thomas N (ed). Wiley-Blackwell.
   - *Handbook of Renal and Pancreatic Transplantation.* Ziring D, Danovitch G, Cohen D (eds). Wiley-Blackwell.

4. Psychological and social aspects of dialysis
   - Living with Kidney Disease: A comprehensive guide for coping with chronic kidney disease. Levy J, Stevens PE. Wiley-Blackwell.
   - Psychosocial Aspects of Chronic Kidney Disease: Exploring the Impact of CKD, Dialysis, and Transplantation on Patients. Agarwal R, Thomas N (eds). Academic Press.

5. Nutrition and dialysis
   - Eating Well with Kidney Failure: A Practical Guide and Cookbook. Thomas M, Thomas N, Lambie H. Class Publishing.

- Renal Diet Cookbook: The Comprehensive Guide for Healthy Kidneys. Jones C. Rockridge Press.

6. Innovations in dialysis
    - Artificial Organs. Nosé Y (ed). Wiley.
    - Telemedicine in the ICU. Vukmir RB. Springer.

7. Medical ethics
    - *The Oxford Handbook of Bioethics.* Steinbock B (ed). Oxford University Press.
    - Medical Ethics: Accounts of Ground-breaking Cases. Pence GE. McGraw-Hill Education.

8. Professional journals
    - Journal of the American Society of Nephrology (JASN)
    - Kidney International
    - American Journal of Kidney Diseases (AJKD)
    - Nephrology Nursing Journal

9. Organisations and associations
    - National Kidney Foundation Official website
    - International Society of Nephrology Official website

10. Online courses and webinars
    - Coursera: Introduction to Kidney Diseases
    - Medscape Nephrology Education

It is important to note that the titles, publishers and links are provided as examples and may need to be updated. Always be sure to consult the most recent editions and check the links for online resources.

• French references and recommended reading

1. General works on nephrology
   * *La Néphrologie en 1001 QCM.* Bourquelot P, Vrtovsnik F (eds). Elsevier Masson.
   * *Nephrology & Therapeutics.* Servais A, Karras A, Boffa JJ, Lang P (eds). Elsevier Masson.

2. Specialisation in dialysis
   * Peritoneal Dialysis for the Nephrologist. Fischbach M, Zaloszyc A (eds). Springer.
   * *L'Hémodialyse à domicile.* Ryckelynck JP, Lobbedez T (eds). Springer.

3. Nephrology nursing care
   * *Nephrology nurse.* CNEPH (Collectif National des Equipes de Prévention en Hémodialyse). Lamarre.

4. Psychological and social aspects of dialysis
   * *Home dialysis.* Bechade C, Lobbedez T, Ryckelynck JP. Elsevier Masson.
   * *L'annonce en néphrologie.* Combe C, Ficheux M, Fouque D. Elsevier Masson.

5. Nutrition and dialysis
   * Dietetics in renal failure. Guérin AS, Allard L. Grancher.
   * *Kidney cooking.* Association France Rein.

6. Innovations in dialysis
   * L'épuration extra-rénale en réanimation. Monchi M, Vinsonneau C (eds). Arnette.

7. Medical ethics
   * Ethical dilemmas in medicine. Hervé C, Moutel G, Duchange N. PUF.

8. Professional journals
   * Nephrology & Therapeutics

- Journal of Nephrology

9. Organisations and associations
- French-speaking Society of Nephrology, Dialysis and Transplantation (SFNDT) <u>Official website</u>
- *France* Rein <u>Official website</u>

10. Online courses and webinars
- <u>MOOC Francophone: kidneyChronic and ëacute</u>
- <u>SFNDT Conferences and Training</u>

It is essential to check that each work is relevant and up-to-date, especially in a constantly evolving medical field. What's more, some titles may have new editions or updated versions.